D0031076

Sleeping Through the Night

Revised Edition

*How Infants, Toddlers, and
Their Parents Can Get
a Good Night's Sleep*

Jodi A. Mindell, Ph.D.

HARPER

NEW YORK • LONDON • TORONTO • SYDNEY

To Scott and Caelie

HarperCollins books may be purchased for educational, business, or sales promotional use. For information please write: Special Markets Department, HarperCollins Publishers Inc., 10 East 53rd Street, New York, NY 10022.

Designed by Ellen Cipriano

Library of Congress Cataloging-in-Publication Data

Mindell, Jodi A.
    Sleeping through the night : how infants, toddlers, and their parents can get a good night's sleep / Jodi A. Mindell.—revised edition.
      p. cm.
    Includes index.
    ISBN 0-06-074256-9
    1. Infants—Sleep. 2. Children—Sleep. 3. Sleep disorders in children. I. Title.
RJ506.S55M54 2005
618.92'8498—dc22

                                            2004054345

10 11 12 WB/RRD 20 19 18 17

This book is designed to give information on various medical conditions, treatments, and procedures for your personal knowledge and to help you be a more informed consumer of medical and health services. It is not intended to be complete or exhaustive, nor is it a substitute for the advice of your physician. You should seek medical care promptly for any specific medical condition or problem your child may have. Under no circumstances should medication of any kind be administered to your child without first checking with your physician.

All efforts have been made to ensure the accuracy of the information contained in this book as of the date published. The authors and the publisher expressly disclaim responsibility for any adverse effects arising from the use or application of the information contained herein.

The names and identifying characteristics of parents and children featured throughout this book have been changed to protect their privacy.

Contents

Part Three: Steps for Success / 149

Part Four: Other Common Sleep Problems / 235

Part Five: "What About Me?":
Adult Sleep and Sleep Problems / 289

Appendices / 339

Index / 351

Acknowledgments

I wish to thank all the families and friends who shared their stories with me, and all of the babies who are now sleeping through the night.

Special thanks are extended to my colleagues, Dr. Judith A. Owens, my compadre in the world of pediatric sleep; Dr. Mary A. Carskadon, who has been a great supporter of my work in pediatric sleep disorders and who has taught me so much; and to my colleagues and the staff at the Sleep Disorders Center at The Children's Hospital of Philadelphia, especially Dr. Raanan Arens and Dr. Alex Mason, who share a weekly sleep clinic with me and help take such great care of our patients. Huge thanks and appreciation to Dr. Lisa Meltzer, the most incredible colleague, who has spent so much time providing assistance and suggestions for this second edition and was always just an e-mail or phone call away for every question imaginable.

Finally, my deepest appreciation to those who have supported this project from the very beginning: my agent, Carol Mann, for her enthusiasm for this book; my editor, Toni Sciarra, for her insightful comments and attention to detail; and, most important, to my husband and best friend, Dr. Scott P. McRobert, for his unwavering support and humor, as well as his amazing talents as a dad. I couldn't have done this book without him. And, lastly, to my daughter, Caelie, who is the light of my life and has taught me all the wonders and joys of being a mom.

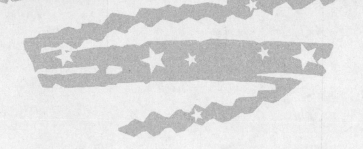

PART ONE

The Basics of Sleep

CHAPTER 1

"Help, My Baby Won't Sleep!": An Introduction to Sleep and Sleep Problems

Lisa and John are at their wits' end. Every night it can take up to two hours to rock their fifteen-month-old son, Ethan, to sleep. He then wakes up at least twice during the night and needs to be rocked back to sleep. Lisa and John frequently fight about what they should do, and at this point they are both too tired to function.

The above scenario describes the situation commonly faced by the parents of infants and toddlers. In fact, this situation is so common that the first question veteran parents ask new parents right after "Is it a boy or a girl?" and "What is her name?" is "Is she sleeping through the night?" Study after study has shown that approximately 25 percent of all young children experience some type of sleep problem. Most of these problems are related to getting to sleep and sleeping through the night.

Sleep, or the lack thereof, is a critical aspect of child rearing. "Good" babies sleep. Most babies don't. As long as everyone gets enough sleep, parents can deal with just about anything during the day. However, when you are awake at 4:00 a.m. facing a screaming baby for the third time that night, all sanity goes out the window. It would try anybody's patience. And what parents resort to as a solution can be incredible: circling the block in their car at 3:30 a.m. wearing their pajamas with mismatched socks, their baby sleeping peacefully in the car seat, trying to imagine how they are going to explain the situation if pulled over by a police officer.

SLEEP—WHAT IS IT?

Everyone sleeps. Humans sleep, toads sleep, monkeys sleep, dogs sleep, and whales sleep. But, surprisingly, we know very little about sleep. Although sleep researchers understand the mechanisms of sleep and what happens to the brain and body when we sleep, we still do not know why we sleep. Some believe sleep has a restorative function. Others believe that we sleep to conserve energy. Still others believe that sleep is adaptive, that it enhances survival. What we do know is that everyone needs to sleep. People cannot function without it. The body craves sleep when too much time has gone by without it. People also don't feel like themselves when they haven't gotten enough sleep. So while we are not exactly sure what sleep is, we do know that we need it.

One aspect of sleep that is well understood is that many people have sleep disorders. Approximately 25–30 percent of adults have a sleep problem, such as insomnia or obstructive sleep apnea, and most adults get too little sleep. Babies and toddlers have sleep problems too. Some are quite serious, such as sleep apnea. Most are just difficult to deal with, such as problems at bedtime or frequent night wakings.

Sleep is a natural process and we all know how to sleep. However, good sleeping habits need to be developed. Bad sleeping habits, especially when trying to fall asleep, are what become problematic for many babies and toddlers. Babies learn to fall asleep under specific circumstances, such as being rocked, being pushed in a stroller, or simply lying in a crib. It is these circumstances that may or may not lead to a baby's sleep problems; that is, many babies develop good sleep habits, whereas other babies develop poor sleep habits. These issues will be addressed more thoroughly throughout this book.

WHY DOESN'T MY BABY SLEEP?

Sleep problems in young children are much more common than you may think. While research studies have consistently shown that between 25 percent and 30 percent of all infants and toddlers have some type of sleep disturbance, a recent National Sleep Foundation *Sleep in America* poll found that almost seven out of ten children (up to age ten) experience some type of sleep problem, and 75 percent of all parents want to change something about their child's sleep. That is a large number of children and families. You are certainly not alone if you have problems with your baby's sleep.

Of course, if your neighbor's baby or your friend's baby sleeps, then you may ask yourself, "Why does my child have a problem?" First of all, and most important, it seems there is a biological predisposition to having sleep problems. This means that some babies are more susceptible to sleep problems than others. Some babies start sleeping through the night within a few weeks of coming home from the hospital and never have any problems with sleep. Other babies, however, never seem to get a good night's sleep. Thus, some babies are born "sleepers" and some babies are not. Some babies have more difficulty learning to fall asleep, are more easily aroused from sleep, and are more sensitive to changes in routines that affect their sleep patterns. I once heard a parent joke that when she ordered her next baby, she was going to check the "sleeper" box. Many parents feel this way.

Some parents blame themselves for their child's sleep problems. Some believe that if they just hadn't rocked him to sleep as an infant, he would be fine. Others feel that they let their child sleep in bed with them for too long, and that is what caused their baby's problems. Unfortunately, the truth is that parents often do play a role in their child's sleep problems. They may inadvertently have instituted poor sleep habits. But a baby's sleep problems are not entirely the parents' fault. The baby also contributes. Many babies who are rocked or nursed to sleep go to sleep quickly and don't wake during the night. It is apparent, then, that the same parenting behavior can lead to sleep problems in some babies and not in others. Parents therefore need to change their behavior only if their baby has a problem sleeping through the night.

PREDICTORS OF SLEEP PROBLEMS

In addition to a biological predisposition, there are certain other factors that place a child at risk for sleep problems. Below are a number of things that can contribute to a baby having a sleep problem.

FIRSTBORN. Firstborns are more at risk for sleep problems. Why? Probably because parents are more anxious with their first child. This is their first time at parenting, and they are usually more concerned about whether they are doing it right or wrong. They tend to be much less tolerant of their child's cries, and they have more time to devote to their first child, including getting up and rocking the baby back to sleep in the middle of the night. Later, when the family is larger, parents tend to set a definite bedtime for the children. When it is bedtime, everyone goes to bed. There are no ifs, ands, or buts about it. And it is rare to have the luxury of rocking later-born children to sleep or nursing them to sleep when you are trying to get everyone into pajamas with teeth brushed and so on.

COLIC OR EAR INFECTIONS. Children with colic or frequent ear infections are much more likely to have sleep problems, primarily because they get into the habit of waking during the night when they aren't feeling well. Then, even when they are feeling better, they may still wake during the night and have difficulty returning to sleep without help from their parents. For the parents, it is difficult to determine whether their baby is still in pain from an ear infection or is just having problems sleeping.

SAME BED OR ROOM. Studies have shown that almost all children who sleep in the same bed or in the same room as their parents wake during the night. Chapter 8 explains why this happens.

BREAST-FEEDING. Breast-fed babies are more likely to fall into the habit of nursing to sleep, and needing to be nursed back to sleep when they naturally awaken during the night. They are also more likely to take longer to sleep through the night. One study found that 52 percent of breast-fed infants, but only 20 percent of bottle-fed infants, wake during the night. A complete discussion of breast-feeding and sleep can be found in Chapter 10.

FOODS. In rare instances foods may be related to sleep problems. For example, milk intolerance may be related to persistent sleeplessness. Some infants with milk intolerance take longer to fall asleep at bedtime, sleep fewer hours, and have more night wakings. Since milk intolerance happens in so few children, it should be suspected only when all the usual causes of sleeplessness have been excluded. Many people believe that the eating of solid foods by infants improves sleep. This is not true. Infants who eat solid foods do not sleep any better than those who do not eat solid foods. Sleeping for longer periods at a stretch is caused by maturation, not changes in diet.

MAJOR CHANGES. Major changes, such as going on a trip, a death in the family, a parent returning to work, an illness, or even a major developmental change, can bring on sleep problems even in babies who were always good sleepers.

AWAKE OR ASLEEP. Studies show that infants who are put to bed already asleep are much more likely to wake during the night than infants who are put in their cribs awake and fall asleep there. The National Sleep Foundation poll found that babies who are put to bed already asleep take longer to fall asleep, are twice as likely to wake during the night, and sleep on average an hour less per night.

So if your baby is asleep before you put her in her crib, she is much less likely to sleep through the night.

IS IT A SLEEP PROBLEM OR IS IT A SLEEP DISORDER?

One question that parents need to ask themselves when faced with a baby who is not sleeping well is whether the problem is a behavioral problem or an indication of a more serious sleep disorder that has an underlying physiological basis. The likelihood is that it is simply a sleep problem that can be managed behaviorally. In rare cases, though, an underlying sleep disorder may be the cause of your child's not sleeping through the night. But even if there is an underlying sleep disrupter, there is often an additional behavioral component. For example, if your child is waking at night because of sleep apnea, she should still be able to put herself back to sleep with no help from you. If she needs you in the middle of the night, she probably also has a sleep problem in addition to the sleep disorder of sleep apnea.

IS IT AN ENVIRONMENTAL PROBLEM?

Another factor that you should consider is whether your child's sleep problems are caused by something in your child's environment. Is your child too cold or too hot during the night? Are loud noises disturbing your child's sleep? Are there spooky shadows on the wall caused by the night-light? Try to change things in your child's bedroom environment that may be causing her problems sleeping. Add room-darkening shades to keep out the morning light. Run a fan or a noise machine to mask household and family noises. If the sleep problems persist, then it is time to look into alternative explanations, namely behavioral issues.

Does Your Child Have a Sleep Disorder?

How do you know if your child has a sleep disorder? The following list of sleep problems may indicate that your child has a sleep disorder:

1. Loud snoring, noisy breathing, or breathing pauses while sleeping.
2. Breathing through his mouth while sleeping.
3. Appearing confused or looking terrified when he awakens during the night.
4. Frequent sleepwalking.
5. Rocking to sleep or head banging when falling asleep or during the night.
6. Complaining of leg pains, "growing pains," or restless legs when trying to fall asleep or during the night.
7. Kicking his legs in a rhythmic fashion while sleeping.
8. Sleeping restlessly.
9. Frequent difficulty falling asleep or staying asleep.
10. Difficulty waking up in the morning or daytime sleepiness.
11. Sleep difficulties leading to daytime behavior problems or irritability.

If your child experiences any of the above, be sure to read about the various sleep disorders described in Chapters 12, 13, and 14. If your child seems to have symptoms of any of these sleep disorders, be sure to discuss the problem with your pediatrician.

IS IT A MEDICAL PROBLEM?

A final factor that you should consider is whether your child's sleep problems are related to a medical problem. The most common medical problem that can disrupt sleep in young children is reflux. Other medical problems include pain as the result of ear infections or teething, as well as asthma or allergies. Consult your child's doctor to be sure that there are no medical problems that are disrupting your child's sleep.

SLEEP PROBLEMS PERSIST

You will often hear "Oh, it is just a stage" or "He'll grow out of it," but this is usually not true for sleep problems. Babies and young children simply do not grow out of most sleep problems. Several studies have found that babies who don't sleep become toddlers who don't sleep and then young children who don't sleep. One study found that 84 percent of children who had sleep problems at a young age continued to have problems three years later. Not only do sleep problems continue, they seem to be one of the most persistent behavioral problems. Studies that looked at many different behavioral problems found that sleep issues were much more likely to persist than other issues, such as temper tantrums or problems with eating. This means that you should not ignore your child's sleep problem. Do something about it now rather than having to deal with it later. It is much easier to deal with sleep problems when your child is an infant and in a crib than later when she is big enough to climb out of a crib or is in a bed. The younger your child is, the easier it will be to teach her to sleep through the night, because the bad sleep habits are less ingrained. But if your child is a bit older, do not despair. It is never too late; it may just take a bit more effort.

THE BENEFITS OF SLEEPING
THROUGH THE NIGHT

Babies who sleep through the night are better rested, happier, and less cranky during the day than babies who don't sleep. Just as you feel terrible the next day after waking several times during the night, so does your baby. There aren't any definitive studies that support these conclusions, but many parents comment on the changes they see when their baby begins to sleep through the night.

Sleeping through the night also helps families. Many studies have observed the negative impact of children's sleep problems on families and the subsequent improvements after the baby is sleeping through the night. More than one marriage has been saved with the onset of a sleeping baby. Parents feel better about themselves as parents and are able to function better once the baby is sleeping. In addition, parents enjoy their children more. After a night of pleading, arguing, and power struggles to get your child to sleep, it is difficult to be enthusiastic about seeing your child in the morning. Happier and better parents make for happier babies.

WHAT WILL BE COVERED IN THIS BOOK

This book provides practical advice and tips on how to get infants and toddlers to sleep through the night. It is geared toward parents of young children, from infancy through three and a half years. Included are steps on how to get babies to fall asleep and sleep through the night, as well as answers to many other common sleep problems.

The method described in this book is designed for parents who want a kinder and gentler approach. This method takes into account a baby's temperament and a family's parenting style, as well as everyday problems that can undo sleep training, such as illness, travel, breast-feeding, toilet training, and babysitters—anything outside the normal routine. This book will help you adjust to and cope with the unexpected, and it will help you succeed in teaching your baby to sleep through the night.

The book is organized into four sections:

Part One (Chapters 1 through 3) provides an introduction to sleep and sleep problems in babies, a basic overview of sleep, and an essential review of basic parenting skills and behavior-management strategies to be used with infants and toddlers.

Part Two (Chapters 4 through 8) helps parents deal with a newborn's first few months and outlines how to establish good sleep habits early to prevent future sleep problems. It outlines how parents can resolve sleep problems and get their infant or toddler to sleep through the night.

Part Three (Chapters 9 through 11) provides the steps for success in sleep training. Coping strategies on how to deal with sleep training are recommended, and common problems that parents encounter are addressed. Ways to resolve obstacles to continued good sleep are presented so that your child will continue to get a good night's sleep.

Part Four (Chapters 12 through 14) introduces other common childhood sleep problems, such as sleep apnea, parasomnias, and nightmares.

Part Five (Chapters 15 and 16) discusses how parents can get the sleep they need, including strategies for improving parents' sleep and common adult sleep disorders.

In addition, there are two appendices:

Appendix A lists recommended bedtime books for infants and toddlers, as well as books for dealing with bedtime fears.

Appendix B presents resources for parents, including organizations and associations that provide additional information on sleep, sudden infant death syndrome (SIDS), breast-feeding, and twins and more groups, as well as general parenting Web sites.

CHAPTER 2

What Is Sleep?

"*Is my baby getting enough sleep?*"

"*When should my one-year-old stop taking morning naps?*"

The information in this chapter about the basics of sleep will help you understand your child's sleep and will be useful when implementing the procedures outlined later for helping your baby sleep through the night.

STAGES OF SLEEP

Sleep is primarily two major states, non-REM and REM. REM stands for rapid-eye-movement sleep. The stages of sleep, as described here, are typical of the sleep of adults. How sleep is different in young children will be discussed later.

Non-REM Sleep

Non-REM sleep is composed of four stages, each with its own distinct features.

STAGE ONE. Stage one sleep occurs when you feel drowsy and start to fall asleep. If the phone rings or something else wakes you, you may not even realize that you have been asleep. Stage one lasts for the first thirty seconds to five minutes of sleep.

Sometimes during stage one sleep a person will awaken with a sudden jerk. This is quite normal. This startling event is actually the result of REM intrusion, meaning that your body has entered REM sleep at the wrong time. The sudden muscle paralysis and onset of dreaming, which are key features of REM sleep, cause you to feel as if you are falling. People who suddenly awaken like this often remember dreaming that they were falling off a cliff or out of an airplane.

STAGE TWO. During stage two sleep, your body moves into a deeper state of sleep. You can still be easily wakened, but you are clearly asleep. The stage two period lasts from ten to forty-five minutes.

STAGES THREE AND FOUR. Stages three and four, known as "deep sleep," are the deepest stages of sleep and a time during which your body experiences the most positive and restorative effects of sleep. A person in either of these two stages has regular, steady breathing and heart rate. For some people, sweating is common during these stages of sleep. You may find that your baby sweats so much that she is soaking wet. This is normal. It is also difficult to be awakened from deep sleep. You may not hear a phone ringing or someone calling your name. When people sleep through earthquakes or major storms, it is because they are in deep sleep. If you do get awakened from deep sleep, you will often be confused, and it will take you a few minutes to respond. Following the first deep sleep period of anywhere from a few minutes to an hour, there is a return to a lighter stage of sleep prior to the first REM period.

REM *Sleep*

REM sleep is distinctly different from non-REM sleep. REM sleep is when you dream. REM sleep is also a very active type of sleep. Both your breathing and heart rate become irregular, although no sweating occurs. The majority of your body, other than the normal functioning of your organs, becomes paralyzed, and all of your muscles become extremely relaxed. Your eyes dart back and forth under your eyelids, hence the term rapid-eye-movement sleep. Some people also experience minor twitching of their hands, legs, or face during REM sleep. (This is sometimes very obvious; you can observe it by watching your dog or cat during REM sleep.) And men usually get erections during REM sleep.

SLEEP CYCLES

Sleep in adults typically occurs in ninety-minute cycles. The first ninety minutes is all non-REM sleep. After ninety minutes, a period of REM sleep will occur, followed by a return to non-REM sleep. After that, about every ninety minutes a REM period will occur. The first REM periods of the night are quite short, lasting just a few minutes. As the night goes on, REM periods increase in length. By early morning much of sleep is REM. This is the reason you are likely to be dreaming when you awaken in the morning. This is also the reason that men may wake with an erection. If you are sleep deprived, the first REM period will be earlier in the night, after only thirty or forty minutes, and more REM sleep will occur. This is the reason your dreams may be much more vivid the first night that you get a good night's sleep after being sleep deprived. People who are sleep deprived will also have more stages three and four sleep on nights they are catching up on their sleep.

Sleep, however, is not totally predictable, and one stage of sleep does not always follow the next. During sleep, the body will move from one stage to another, not necessarily in any particular order or in any logical fashion. In general, your body will cycle sequentially through all the stages of sleep, but not always. Some nights you may never have any stage three or four sleep. Other nights you will have a great deal.

STRUCTURE OF SLEEP IN INFANTS AND YOUNG CHILDREN

Like everything else that changes as you grow, sleep changes too. Sleep in infants is dramatically different from sleep in children, adolescents, and adults. Infant sleep patterns begin to develop in the uterus, before birth. A fetus of six or seven months' gestation experiences REM sleep, with non-REM sleep beginning shortly afterward. By the end of the eighth month of gestation, sleep patterns are well established.

The Early Months

ACTIVE VERSUS QUIET SLEEP. Instead of using the classifications of REM and non-REM sleep, as is done with adults, researchers classify the sleep of a newborn infant as either active or quiet. During active (REM) sleep, infants are quite mobile. They may move their arms or legs, cry or whimper, and their eyes may be partly open. Their breathing is irregular, and their eyes may dart back and forth under their eyelids. During quiet (non-REM) sleep, infants are behaviorally quiescent. Their breathing is regular, and they lie very still. They may, however, have an occasional startle response or make sucking movements with their mouths. The quiet (non-REM) sleep in infants does not have the four stages of non-REM sleep seen in adults. It is not until about six months that babies develop the four distinct stages of non-REM sleep.

In addition, an infant's sleep is different in structure from that of adults. For example, about 50 percent of the sleep of newborns is active (REM) sleep, whereas REM constitutes only about 20–25 percent of adult sleep. As in adults, active (REM) sleep is cyclical, but in comparison to the ninety-minute cycle of adults, infant cycles are sixty minutes. Also, infants may immediately have an active (REM) period upon falling asleep, which is unusual for adults to experience.

Quiet (non-REM) sleep in infants is also different from non-REM sleep in adults. First, as mentioned above, infants do not have the characteristic four stages experienced by adults. Also, quiet (non-REM) sleep accounts for a smaller proportion of total sleep time—50 percent in infants rather than almost 75 percent in adults. These differences between infants' and adults' sleep patterns quickly dissipate. By three months of age, the sleep stages of infants begin to resemble those of adults. For example, short bursts of rapid brain activity, known as "stage two spindle activity," occur by three or four months. Also, another aspect of sleep, "spontaneous K complexes," which are characterized by large, slow brain waves during sleep, develops at six months. Other changes include a decrease in REM sleep and an increase in non-REM sleep so that by six months of age REM sleep accounts for 30 percent of the time sleeping and non-REM for 70 percent of the time—more like adult sleep.

BABIES ARE NOT QUIET SLEEPERS. As anyone who has watched a baby sleep knows, babies are not quiet sleepers. Babies will smile, sigh, squeak, coo, moan, groan, and whimper in their sleep. Toddlers and young children will sigh, talk, mumble, and grumble. It is all perfectly normal. Don't worry that your child is not getting good solid sleep if he seems to be active during sleep.

The Later Months

By six months of age, the full spectrum of non-REM and REM sleep occurs. However, the percentage of time spent in each stage is still different from that in adults, as is the length of the sleep cycle. Not until your child is three or four years old will her sleep resemble an adult's sleep. Young children continue to spend more time in REM sleep, and during non-REM sleep they go into deep, stage four sleep faster. For example, if your child falls asleep in the car, she may be in deep sleep within ten minutes. Upon arriving home you can bring her in the house, change her, and put her to bed without her ever stirring.

After about an hour of deep sleep, your child will typically have a brief arousal. Most children will simply move or grimace briefly. Other children will have a more pronounced arousal, even to the point of sleepwalking or having a sleep terror (see Chapter 13 for a full description). After this arousal, your child will return to deep sleep. An arousal may also happen after a period of REM sleep, but it will be very different. During this type of arousal your child will be awake and alert, as always occurs after waking from REM sleep. This will be the time of night when your child may call out to you because he needs you to help him go back to sleep. These are normal night wakings. They are problematic only if your baby can't go back to sleep on his own. You may then need to rock or nurse him back to sleep. Dealing with these types of night wakings is covered in Chapter 6.

SLEEP PATTERNS

Another difference between infants' and adults' sleep is how their sleep patterns are organized. Infants have polyphasic sleep periods, meaning that they have many sleep periods throughout the day, whereas adults typically have only one sleep period lasting about eight hours (although there are many adults who continue to nap). In the beginning, your baby will be sleeping in two- to four-hour blocks throughout the day. By eight weeks of age, your baby will begin to have a clear diurnal/nocturnal sleep pattern; that is, she will begin to be awake more during the day and sleep more at night. As she gets older, your baby's sleep will begin to consolidate—she will begin to sleep fewer times throughout the day but for longer periods.

Finally, it is important to understand that every infant displays a unique sleeping pattern. The information presented here provides broad generalizations drawn from the behavior of hundreds of infants. However, your child's sleep pattern may very well be different. Some newborns sleep through the night immediately, whereas the sleep of others does not consolidate for several months. In all ways, the sleep patterns of infants are as different and varied as those seen in adults.

INTERNAL CLOCK

Parents often struggle with getting their child to establish a sleep pattern during the day, basically getting them to fall asleep at the same times throughout the day. Helping a child fall asleep quickly and at roughly the same time every day is based on two key things. The first is what time a child wakes up. What time a child wakes up will set his clock for the day. It's a bit like pushing the start button on a timer. When the timer goes off, it will then be time to fall asleep. Your baby's "start" button in the morning will not only set naptimes, but it will set bedtime, too. So you can't control what time your child falls asleep, but you can definitely control what time your child wakes up.

The second factor is keeping to a consistent daytime and evening schedule by putting your child to bed at close to the same time every day. Again, this will help set your child's internal clock and train his body to be sleepy at the same times every day.

NAPPING

Although almost all babies nap, it may take a few months before your baby establishes a napping schedule. Between three and six months of age, a little more than half of all babies are taking three or more naps per day; the rest are taking two naps a day. Between six and nine months most children (nearly 60 percent) are taking only two naps per day, a morning nap and an afternoon nap, usually at set times. Most babies move to one nap a day by eighteen months. Most toddlers continue to nap until they are three years old, with many children starting to give up naps after their third birthday. Not until a child is between three and six years old will all sleep occur at one time: during the night. Remember, though, every child is different. Some children will stop napping by age three, while others continue to need a nap until they are six.

Naps are very beneficial. Children who nap have longer attention spans and are less fussy than their nonnapping counterparts. Some parents, concerned about their child's nighttime sleeping habits, try to get their child to sleep more at night by depriving their child of a daytime nap. This is not effective and may in fact be detrimental, since children need naps. Also, evidence shows that keeping children up during the day does not help them sleep more at night. Rather, for younger children, eliminating naps can backfire because the more overtired a child becomes, the more difficulty he will have going to sleep at night.

Basically, sleep begets sleep. The better a child sleeps during the day, the better he will sleep at night—and the better he sleeps at night, the better he will sleep during the day. After age five, however, eliminating afternoon naps can help get your child to bed earlier in the evening.

It is best to have your child nap in the same place that she sleeps at night on days that she is napping at home. In this way sleep will be strongly associated with her crib or bed, which is important to help your child sleep through the night. Napping on the couch or in the car may also cause naps to be shorter because your child will be awakened by the activities of others or when the car stops. A set naptime in a set place will ensure that your child gets the proper sleep that she needs. The best times for naps are midmorning for morning naps and early afternoon for afternoon naps. Don't let your child sleep past 4:00 in the afternoon, or she may have a difficult time falling asleep at bedtime.

If your child is watched by a caregiver during the day, whether at home or in another setting, make naptimes consistent. Try to have your child nap at the same time every day, no matter who is caring for her. Also, discuss with your caregiver the latest time for your child to sleep in the afternoon so that your child can fall asleep easily at an appropriate time at night.

For lots more information on naps and dealing with naptime problems, see Chapter 7.

WAKING DURING THE NIGHT

Waking during the night is a normal part of sleep. Everyone does it—babies wake, children wake, adolescents wake, and adults wake. Many people, though, don't even know that they do it. They may wake for anywhere from a few seconds to a couple of minutes, and return immediately to sleep. The human body is programmed to do this. In fact, studies show that a person has to be awake for at least three to five minutes to be aware of waking. So if you remember waking up last night, then you know that you must have been up for at least three minutes.

Most infants fall back to sleep on their own after waking at night. These infants are called "self-soothers." Most parents of self-soothers never even know their baby was awake several times during the night. In contrast, infants known as "signalers" cannot return to sleep on their own after waking during the night. Parents of "signalers" know when their baby is awake at night. These babies need help falling back to sleep—and they signal this need by crying.

There have been many studies of night wakings in young children. By six months of age, almost all infants are physiologically capable of sleeping through the night and no longer need nighttime feedings; however, about one-third to one-half continue to awaken at night. Night waking becomes more problematic again between the ages of six and nine months. This is likely due to physiological changes and to other developmental issues, such as developmental milestones (it is much more fun to practice standing than it is to sleep!). Estimates indicate that 25–50 percent of six- to twelve-month-olds wake during the night, and 25 percent of one-year-olds continue to do so.

PULLING IT ALL TOGETHER—BY AGE

How much sleep your child needs will change as she gets older. Also, different sleep issues will occur at different ages. Recommended hours of sleep are shown in the table. The table on page 23 was developed by members of the National Sleep Foundation's pediatric task force, which I chair. Note that the averages presented (as well as the recommended hours noted below within each section) are simply that, averages. Some children will sleep two hours more or two hours less. Also, recent research has shown that the greatest individual differences in sleep need occur in the first year of life. Our sleep needs become more and more similar as we get older.

The figure on page 24 presents the amount of sleep that parents report children are getting in the United States. These data come from the 2004 National Sleep Foundation's *Sleep in America* poll (I also chaired this poll), a telephone survey of almost 1,500 parents or caregivers of children ages ten and under. Note, however, that half of all parents (50 percent) reported that their child was not

Recommended Total Hours of Sleep

Age Group	Age	Recommended Hours
Infants	2 months to 12 months	14–15 hours
Toddlers	12 months to 3 years	12–14 hours
Preschoolers	3 years to 6 years	11–13 hours
School-aged	6 years to 12 years	10–11 hours
Adolescents	12 years to 18 years	8.5–9.5 hours

Source: *National Sleep Foundation pediatric task force*

getting enough sleep; so be careful not to use this information as recommended hours of sleep.

Newborns (0 to Two Months)

A newborn typically sleeps anywhere from ten to eighteen hours a day. Sleep is equally spaced throughout the day, with no clear differentiation between daylight hours and nighttime hours. A bottle-fed baby will typically sleep three to five hours at a time, whereas a breast-fed baby will sleep two to three hours. Some babies, though, will sleep for even shorter times. For parents, who are used to sleeping anywhere from six to nine hours at a stretch, suddenly being on their baby's schedule can be very difficult. Your baby may be getting lots of sleep, but you aren't.

By six to eight weeks of age, expect to put your child down to sleep after she has been up for about two hours. That is about a baby's limit at this age for how long she will be awake and stay happy and alert. If you wait too long after two hours, she may become overtired and have a more difficult time going to sleep. So try to put her down to sleep before she gets upset. Start to look for signs that your baby is getting tired, such as rubbing her eyes,

Average Number of Hours Children Sleep

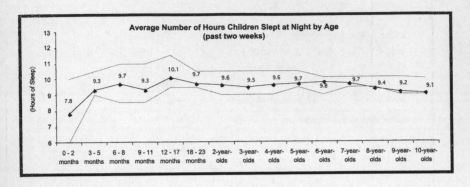

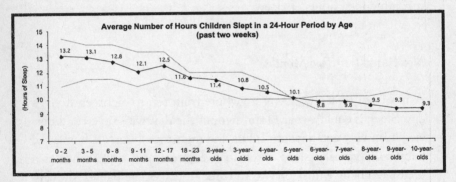

Source: 2004 National Sleep Foundation *Sleep in America* poll

✦ Dark line indicates average number of hours
✦ Top line indicates 75th percentile
✦ Bottom line indicates 25th percentile

pulling on her ear, or getting slight circles under her eyes. The minute that you see the sign, put her down. Don't wait too long, because if you miss your window of opportunity, getting her down will be a struggle.

SLEEP ISSUES. Sleep issues are common in this early period, mostly because parents have a difficult time with their lack of sleep.

✦ **Day/night reversal.** Many newborns in the first few weeks have their days and nights switched, sleeping like a baby all day but awake and active at night. Parents should increase their baby's activity during the day (especially waking for feedings) and keep lights dim at night. For more suggestions on how to deal with day/night reversal, see Chapter 4.

✦ **Safe sleep practices.** Information on crib safety is presented in Chapter 5 and tips on decreasing the risk of sudden infant death syndrome (SIDS) can be found in Chapter 12. Be sure and put your baby down to sleep on his or her back.

✦ **Parents' need for sleep.** Parents need to ensure that they get the sleep they need. Some studies indicate that sleep deprivation may be a risk factor for postpartum depression.

Infants (Two to Twelve Months)

As infants get older, their sleep begins to consolidate, and they begin to sleep less. Babies begin to sleep for longer stretches at night

---

Sleep Tips for Newborns

✦ Learn your baby's signs of being sleepy.
✦ Follow your baby's cues, as your newborn may prefer to be rocked or fed to sleep. By three months, however, begin to establish good sleep habits.
✦ Place your baby on his or her back to sleep.
✦ Encourage nighttime sleep.
✦ Make sleep a family priority.

beginning around eight weeks. This will occur earlier for some babies and later for others. Two-month-olds need about fourteen to fifteen hours of sleep, getting about nine to ten hours at night and five hours of sleep during the day. By one year, they need a total of about fourteen hours of sleep, getting eleven to twelve hours at night and two and a half hours during the day.

Around three to four months, your baby will start going to bed earlier at night. When it comes to waking at night, the rule of thumb is that by six months all babies are physically capable of sleeping through the night, with most being able to do so at a younger age. Babies, however, who are "sleeping through the night," wake for brief periods during the night but can put themselves back to sleep. Thus, many parents who assume their child is sleeping for periods of ten to twelve hours continuously may be inaccurate in their assessment. Their child may actually be waking for brief periods of time without disrupting anyone.

When your baby is between six and nine months, she may begin to have sleep problems even if she has never had them before. These sleep problems usually coincide with cognitive and motor development, not with a growth spurt. Parents who think their baby is going through a growth spurt often decide their baby is waking during the night because she is hungry. This is likely not true. Try to avoid feeding her during the night. You will just prolong the sleep problem and make it worse. Your baby can get all the nutrition she needs during the day. If your baby is going to bed between 8:00 and 9:00 p.m. and all of a sudden she begins to waken during the night, you'll find that, surprisingly, she's much more likely to sleep through the night if you move her bedtime earlier by a half hour or more. It really works. Try it.

Babies shift from taking three to four naps at two months of age to taking two naps by a year of age. Each nap will last anywhere from thirty minutes to two hours. Most young babies are ready to nap two hours after they last woke up. Many babies take several short naps throughout the day, each lasting only thirty to forty-five minutes. Other babies will take two longer naps. Either pattern is perfectly fine.

SLEEP ISSUES. The most common sleep issues that parents face are night wakings (see Chapter 6) and naptime problems (see Chapter 7).

- ✦ **Night wakings.** The most common sleep problem that parents of infants struggle with is nighttime awakenings. All infants and children naturally awaken two to six times throughout the night. Those babies who can soothe themselves to sleep (self-soothers) will quickly return to sleep on their own. On the other hand, those babies who are unable to soothe themselves to sleep (signalers) may need to be rocked, nursed, or given a bottle to return to sleep. See Chapter 6 on how to help your baby sleep through the night.

- ✦ **Nighttime feedings.** Most babies no longer need night-time feedings after six months of age. Check with your child's doctor to be sure whether or not your child continues to need these feedings. Breast-fed babies are more likely to awaken at night for feedings and may take longer to sleep through the night.

- ✦ **Naptime problems.** Many parents struggle with naps. Some of these babies also don't sleep through the night, whereas others are champion nighttime sleepers. Nap issues can be very frustrating to parents, especially if they feel that they spend their entire day trying to get their baby to take a nap.

Toddlers (Twelve Months to Three Years)

Toddlers need between twelve and fourteen hours of sleep total. Usually, toddlers sleep eleven to twelve hours at night and another one to three hours during the day. At one year your toddler is probably still taking two naps per day. By eighteen months, however, most toddlers have given up their morning nap and are napping only once a day for one and a half to two hours (see Chapter 7 for information on transitioning to one nap a day). Some toddlers do continue morning naps until the age of two, so don't force your child into a once-a-day nap schedule because you think that she is too old to nap twice a day. Relish the continued peace and quiet. There will probably be a period of time when one nap is too little and two naps are too much. There are different ways to deal with this transition period. One choice is to alternate one-nap and two-nap days, depending on the prior night's sleep. Another alternative is to put your child to bed earlier in the evening on one-nap days. Most toddlers go to bed between 7:00 and 9:00 p.m. and wake between 6:30 and 8:00 a.m.

SLEEP ISSUES. Sleep problems continue to be common with toddlers, with 25–30 percent of parents of toddlers reporting sleep concerns. Night wakings are experienced by 15–20 percent of toddlers, and resisting going to bed is also very common. Nighttime fears and nightmares also start to develop later in the toddler years.

- **Night wakings.** Night wakings continue to be the number one reported problem with toddlers. Toddlers usually wake up at night and need their parents' help to get back to sleep for the same reason as infants. See Chapter 6 on how to help a toddler sleep through the night.
- **Bedtime struggles.** Some children also start to resist bedtime between the ages of two and three, while others get out of their crib or bed at night. These issues are discussed in Chapters 6 and 10.
- **Naps.** Some parents continue to struggle with naps during the toddler years. In addition, many parents start to face new naptime issues when their child gets closer to three years. Naptime issues are discussed in Chapter 7.
- **Moving from a crib to a bed.** During this age span, most children move from a crib to a bed. Chapter 11 provides tips on how to make this transition seamless.
- **Transitional objects.** Having a "lovey" becomes increasingly important during the toddler years. A blanket, a stuffed animal, or a doll can help a toddler settle down and fall asleep on her own. Chapter 5 discusses the benefits of a transitional object and ways you may be able to foster one in your child. Remember, not all children take to a lovey.
- **Nighttime fears and nightmares.** Many two- to three-year-olds start to have fears—of the dark, of monsters, or of being separated from you. These fears are common and are part of normal development. Ways to deal with these common fears and nightmares are discussed in Chapter 14.

Preschoolers (Three to Six Years)

Older children are not a focus of this book but will be discussed here so you know what to expect. At these ages most children are still going to sleep between 7:00 and 9:00 at night and waking between 6:30 and 8:00 in the morning. Preschoolers need between 11 and 13 hours per day, with most sleep occurring at night. Most three- and four-year-olds are still taking afternoon naps, with most children giving up their naps by the age of five. Don't force your child to give up naps too early because of nursery school schedules or other planned activities. Some children need their naps, and you will pay the price if you ignore this need. If your child was a good sleeper, he probably still is, and it is rare for new sleep problems to develop after age three. Children of this age are excellent at stalling bedtime, however, and have learned to ask for another drink of water, to tell you just one more time that they love you, or to need to go to the potty incessantly.

GETTING ENOUGH SLEEP

Make sure that your baby gets plenty of sleep! Even if it is not a priority for you, sleep should be a priority for your baby. Although we don't know the exact purpose of sleep, we know that it is important and vital for babies. Without it, your baby will not develop as he should.

As part of the plan to ensure that your baby gets plenty of sleep, a reasonable bedtime is essential. Most babies and children, from the age of three months until at least ten years, need no less than ten to twelve hours of uninterrupted sleep at night. An appropriate baby bedtime is between 7:30 and 8:30. Some young children even go to bed by 6:30 or 7:00. If you are keeping your baby up late at night because you work during the day and you are also waking him early to get him to day care, he is not getting enough sleep. Don't deny your baby what he needs based on your needs or your schedule. Part of being a good parent is ensuring your child's well-being. Getting adequate sleep is part of that well-being.

Reminders ───────────────────────────────────

- ✦ Sleep is composed of two major states, non-REM and REM sleep.
- ✦ Infant sleep patterns, which are different from the patterns of adults, begin to develop before birth.
- ✦ Newborns sleep many times throughout the day, but by six months most babies have a predictable sleep pattern consisting of a long night's sleep plus a morning and afternoon nap.
- ✦ Naps are important and are independent of nighttime sleep.
- ✦ All babies wake during the night. By the age of six months, however, self-soothers can return to sleep on their own while signalers need help to fall back to sleep.
- ✦ Babies need lots of sleep.

CHAPTER 3

"Please Be Good": Managing Behavior

Theresa often gets frustrated with her son, Andrew. Everyone tells her that it is just the "terrible twos," but this doesn't make her feel better. She can't get Andrew to stay still for anything, he is always hitting and biting the other children at day care, and she can't leave him alone for a moment because he inevitably breaks something. She feels that she spends all her time with Andrew pleading with him to "please be good."

Before you can begin to implement the suggestions made in this book, you need to understand the basic principles of behavior management. The concepts discussed in this chapter are universal to all behavior problems, whether it is refusing to lie down for diaper changes, throwing food, or having temper tantrums in grocery stores. These concepts are also applicable to sleep issues. Sleep problems and the behaviors surrounding sleep are not uniquely different from other behavioral problems parents encounter. Sleep issues are just a bit more complex. This chapter addresses the ways to get babies and toddlers to do what you want and how to stop them from doing what you don't want.

When you think about modifying your child's behavior, you want to focus on increasing good behavior and decreasing bad behavior. If you think of it this way, you will keep in mind your ultimate goal: having a well-behaved child. Your role is to be a parent, not a disciplinarian or a judge and jury. Parenting means teaching your child right from wrong, teaching him how to be good and how not to be bad.

GET YOUR CHILD TO DO WHAT YOU WANT

There are many ways to get your child to do what you want. A number of tried-and-true methods are provided here.

Reinforcement

Reinforcement, otherwise known as rewards, is the best way to get your child to do what you want. Reinforcement increases good behavior. Praise your child for doing the right thing, be it eating properly with a fork or being quiet in the library. Don't feel awkward or embarrassed to do this, even in public places. Reinforcement will help your child to know right from wrong. Reinforcement works.

WHAT DOES YOUR CHILD LIKE? It may sound easy to reward a child, but every child likes something different. You need to figure out what it is that your child likes and what he doesn't like. What is fun and exciting for one child can be scary and upsetting for another. Does your child like his feet tickled, or would he rather play peekaboo? Your child may have a favorite toy or favorite sound that you make that always makes him laugh. Some children love to roughhouse and be thrown up in the air, while others would become scared and instantly cry. Some children love to cuddle. You'll need to spend time simply observing your child. What does he like? What gets him excited?

You will have noticed differences between babies, beginning at a very young age, in terms of what they like. Some parents find that a swing is their savior. Their child is in bliss the moment he is put in the swing. Other parents find that a swing is a waste of money: their child just cries every time he is put in it. When your child is young, it can be easier to distinguish his likes and dislikes. As a newborn, he will have basically two states. One involves crying when he doesn't like something, and the other involves being calm when he does like something. As your child gets older, his responses to things become more complex, and whether he likes or dislikes something will be more difficult to distinguish. You must spend time with your child in order to learn what he does and does not enjoy.

PRAISE. There is a lot to be said for praise. Praise is a highly effective behavior-management tool. We don't spend nearly enough time praising children. Think about how happy it makes you when someone tells you that you look good or appreciates something you have done. And people often complain that their partners don't say nearly enough nice things about them. So don't give your child short shrift. Take the time to tell him he is good. Mention his good points. Tell him how proud you are of him. A good rule of thumb is to praise your child at least three or four times for every time you tell your child he is doing something wrong.

Some argue that you are spoiling your child if you praise him too much. Others say not to praise a child or give him a treat for doing something that he should be doing anyway, such as cleaning up his room or behaving at the dinner table. There is no such thing as too much praise or too much love. Your child will prosper when encouraged to do the right thing.

SPEND TIME. Another excellent way to teach your child how to behave is to spend time with him to demonstrate appropriate behavior. For example, coloring together will show him an acceptable behavior. Also, during your time together, comment on what he is doing. While playing with blocks together say, "Wow! You put the blue block on top of the yellow block." Again, this is a way of showing him that you approve of what he is doing.

TREATS (OTHERWISE KNOWN AS BRIBERY). Bribery gets bad press. At times it can be worthwhile to bribe your child. "If you clean up your toys, we can play outside." "If you are quiet in the store, we'll go get pizza." Now, the important thing about using bribery is to give your child the treat only if he really did what he was supposed to do. Going to get pizza even if he misbehaved in the store will teach him that no matter what he does, he gets what he wants. That is not the way it works in the real world, and it shouldn't be the way it works in your child's world.

When establishing positive consequences for behavior, your child's appropriate behavior must be clearly spelled out. "Be good" doesn't mean much to a child. Rather, "Stay with Daddy," "Be quiet," or "Don't touch anything" is much clearer. "Get ready for school" is not specific enough. It is better to tell your child the specific things that need to be done, such as "Get dressed," "Eat breakfast," "Get your knapsack," or "Put on your coat."

The consequences should also fit the behavior. In the work world, you would never get paid ten thousand dollars for walking down the hall to mail some letters. On the other hand, you wouldn't get five dollars for working forty hours. The same should be true for your child. Small behaviors should get small rewards, and big behaviors should get big rewards. You can also establish short-term goals and long-term goals. The general rule is the younger the child, the shorter the goal; that is, for young children, little time should pass between the good behavior and getting rewarded. For using the potty each time, give your child a treat. After a week of using the potty consistently, get her that toy she wants. Do the same thing for other behaviors. Establish daily and weekly goals.

Give Acceptable Choices

Young children have little control over their lives. They eat when they are told to eat, sleep when they are told to sleep, and go for a ride when they are told to get in the car. But young children, like most people, like to have some control over their lives. So whenever possible, give your child choices. It is best to give only two choices, three at the most, or else it will be overwhelming (let your child pick from two pairs of pajamas, not five or six). Of course, only give him choices that are acceptable to you. Rather than asking, "Do you want to go to bed now?" ask, "Do you want to go to bed now or in five minutes?" This way your child feels that he has some control, and you get your child to bed. "Do you want carrots or peas?" ensures that your child eats some type of vegetable.

Don't Ask Questions When You Don't Mean It

Don't ask a question when you really mean to tell your child to do something. Questions allow your child to say no. Think about it. "Do you want to put your toys away?" "Do you want to take a nap?" If you are a child, the obvious answer is no. You then have no choice but to give in to your child's response or follow up by telling your child that he has to do it anyway. When your child really doesn't have a choice, don't provide him with one. Give directions as directions, not as questions.

Make Reasonable Rules

Another downfall for parents is setting unreasonable rules. Unreasonable rules are difficult or impossible for a child to follow. Reasonable rules take an appropriate amount of time and are doable. A reasonable rule for a one-year-old would be to put his jacket on a chair. It takes little time and can be done by a child of that age. A reasonable rule for a two-and-a-half-year-old would be to get his socks and shoes. An unreasonable rule for a two-year-old would be to go upstairs, pick out clothes, get dressed, and brush his teeth. This direction is likely to be beyond the capabilities of a child that age. It also has too many embedded directions. By the time your child gets upstairs, he may not be able to remember all the other things that need to be done. Overwhelmed, he will sit down to play. You will be angry when, ten minutes later, you find him playing contentedly with his trucks. He is not being disobedient; it was just that the tasks were too much for him.

Your rules should also be very specific. "Clean up your room" is not specific. Does this mean put all the toys away, or does it mean to dust all the furniture as well? Also, what you think is clean and what your child thinks is clean are probably two very different things. A better rule is "Put all your toys in the toy box." It is specific and clear, and everyone will know if it has been done. Being told to "be good" when walking in a store is not clear. What in the world does "being good" mean? Rather, tell your child, "I want you to be quiet, hold my hand, and not touch anything while we are in the store." Your child will now know what is expected of him, and it is clear what he is supposed to do.

Have Few Rules

Expect to be tested. Children will test most requests made of them. They will make sure that this is a real rule about which you will be consistent. There are many ways that children test rules. They will break the rule, break part of the rule, argue, plead, cry, scream, or have a temper tantrum. They are not doing this to be belligerent. They are doing this to make sure that the rule stands. Once you expect a child to test you, you will be much better prepared for it and will not feel that it is a personal attack.

It is therefore best to have few rules. If you were to keep count of how many times you told your child to do something over the course of one day, you would be astounded. Between your child testing the rules and your not having enough energy to follow through on every request, it is impossible to expect your child to be perfectly behaved all the time. The best tactic is to make as few requests as possible. The best place to start is with one rule for yourself: Don't have rules for every single problem. It just won't work.

STOP YOUR CHILD FROM DOING
WHAT YOU DON'T WANT

Much of the time you will be focusing on how to get your child to stop doing something that you don't like, be it climbing out of his high chair or hitting another child. This section talks about how to shift your child from behaving badly to being well-behaved. First, though, a discussion on punishment is important because this is often the first choice made by many parents when faced with a misbehaving child.

Punishment

The first reaction of most parents is to punish their children when they do something wrong. This punishment can entail yelling, taking away privileges, spanking, or sending a child to his room. At that particular moment, punishment seems like the right solution to the problem, but it typically doesn't work in the long run.

PUNISHMENT RARELY WORKS. Punishment is not very effective in changing children's behavior—or anyone's behavior, for that matter. Think about yourself and punishment. Imagine yourself driving down the highway. The speed limit is fifty-five miles per hour. All the cars around you seem to be going sixty-five miles per hour or more. Why do they do this? Every driver knows that there is a chance of getting a ticket and being fined a large amount. That doesn't seem to deter speeding. Imagine yourself now driving sixty-five miles per hour. You just passed Exit 11, and you get pulled over by a police officer and given a ticket for $120. After much grumbling, you pay it. Will you speed again? Sure you will, but likely not around Exit 11. That is how people behave. If they do change their behavior following punishment, it is usually specific to those particular circumstances.

PUNISHMENT DOESN'T TEACH APPROPRIATE BEHAVIOR. At some point parents make the daunting discovery that they are the ones who have to teach their child everything: how to dress herself, how to make a phone call, how to behave in a library, and so on. It can be quite intimidating. Punishment will only teach a child what not to do; it doesn't teach what to do. Randy realized this when he was dealing with his daughter, Melissa, who was coloring on the furniture. The first time he caught her coloring on the table, he yelled at her. The next time, Melissa colored on the kitchen counter. He took her crayons away for the afternoon. Later, when Melissa then colored on the wall, he sent her to sit in the "naughty chair."

Obviously, Melissa wasn't getting the message. Punishment wasn't working. Melissa needed to be taught that coloring should be done only on paper. As obvious as that may be to an adult, it is not obvious to a three-year-old. Melissa needed to be taught exactly what was the right thing to do.

SPANKING DOESN'T USUALLY WORK. Punishment that involves spanking or hitting is even less effective. Often spanking or hitting is done in response to your child doing something truly bad, such as biting or hitting. By spanking your child for this behavior, you have taught him that hitting is sometimes okay and that hitting is an effective way to stop someone from doing something you don't like. You are simply modeling a behavior that you don't want your child to do. Imagine the confusion: you are spanking your child and saying that he shouldn't hit anyone else. Your child will learn more by your actions than by your words.

PUNISHMENT RARELY LASTS. Another disadvantage to punishment is that it works only in the short run. Punishment is not a long-term solution. It may be effective for a few minutes or for the afternoon, but it won't change your child's behavior the next day or the next week. This is because punishment doesn't teach your child a correct replacement behavior.

DON'T USE YOUR CHILD'S CRIB, BED, OR BEDROOM FOR PUNISHMENT. Another mistake that many parents make is to put a child in his crib or room as a consequence of bad behavior. This is not good because you don't want your child to associate his crib or bed with punishment. Your child's crib is obviously a convenient place to put him when he misbehaves. It puts him in time-out, gets him away from you, and ensures that he will be safe. Unfortunately, it can lead to more problems. Your child will think that he is being punished when you put him to bed at night.

Instead, you should have a special place, such as a "naughty chair" or a certain room, where he must go when he is acting up. Some parents have found it effective to set up a playpen in another room. This way they have a safe place that is not the crib to put a misbehaving child.

Saying No

Saying no can be hard for parents to do, but it is something they must do often. Some ways to say no are better than others. First, when you say no, mean it. Say it in a firm voice and follow through. Second, be calm. The calmer you are, the more your child will know that you mean it. If you lose control, your child will lose control. Last, be consistent! If you say no the first and second times, be sure to say no the ninth time.

When telling your child she did something wrong, always be sure to comment on your child's behavior, not on her character. Be sure you make clear that you are upset that your daughter threw her cup, not that you think she is a bad person. Don't tell her, "You are bad." Tell her, "Don't throw your cup." Be sure to tell her that what she did was bad, not that she is bad. Telling your child that she is bad, lazy, worthless, or stupid can have many negative consequences. First, and most important, it affects a child's self-esteem. A child's evaluation of herself depends in large part on what her parents think: "If Mom or Dad thinks I am bad, then I must be bad (or lazy or stupid)." Children need as much confidence as they can get to do well in life. Another reason that this tactic doesn't work is that it will become a self-fulfilling prophecy. If you tell your child that she is lazy, why should she bother to put her toys away? In her mind it is not going to change your opinion of her. Also, a child will feel that she can't change something that is part of who she is, but she can change her behavior. So let your child know that you are frustrated because she gets dressed so slowly, not that she is slow.

Ignoring

Ignoring bad behavior is a powerful tool. Much bad behavior is done to get your attention. If the end result is to get your attention, then change the consequences. Ignore the behavior instead.

Think about what frequently happens when a parent is on the phone. The parent is talking to someone else and not paying any attention to the child. This is a time when many children act up. Why do they act up? To get their parent's attention. Imagine yourself in that situation. The phone rings. You go to answer it, leaving your child playing quietly with her building blocks. It is your close friend whom you haven't spoken to in days. You settle in to hear her latest story when you hear a huge crash from the next room. You tell your friend to hold on and go to see what happened. Your daughter has pulled all the videotapes off the shelf. You put her back near her blocks and tell her that you are on the phone and that she needs to play quietly. You go back to the phone, and your friend continues her story. Within a minute you hear another crash and a thunk. You tell your friend that you'd better go and save your belongings, and you'll call her back later. Upon entering the living room again you see that your daughter has pulled all the books off the shelf too. You yell at her and sit down on the floor to help pick up the books and videos.

What has your child just learned from this situation? She has learned that if she misbehaves, you will get off the phone. If she had continued to sit quietly and play with blocks, you would have remained on the phone, ignoring her. She got what she wanted: your attention. And you had to stop doing what you were doing.

In many situations the correct response is to ignore your child's bad behavior. Ignoring the bad behavior will make it go away. In psychological terms this is called "extinction." It works. Obviously, you cannot ignore your child's behavior if she is putting herself in danger or is about to destroy something. In those cases you must get her or your belongings out of harm's way and then go back to ignoring her. She'll get the message.

You must also understand, however, that when you start to ignore a behavior, the behavior will often get worse before it gets better. This is your child's way of saying, "I mean it. Pay attention to me!" If you persist, your efforts will be rewarded. So if your child is singing loudly to get your attention while you are talking to someone else, ignore it. You can take a moment and tell him that it would make you happy if he stopped, but go right back to your conversation. When the singing doesn't work to get your attention, your child will stop. Then praise him for stopping the singing. Ignoring bad behavior can be difficult to do, but it will pay off in the long run.

Time-out

Time-out is a highly effective method for managing your child's behavior. Time-out involves placing your child someplace where he must sit quietly for a few moments after he has misbehaved. This can be a very good way to deal with your child's bad behavior while remaining calm yourself. A child being sent to a certain room or being made to sit on the stairs or in a chair are all forms of time-out. And though it may seem to be a type of punishment, it is not the same as being yelled at or being spanked. Best of all, it can be done almost anywhere.

Time-out sounds a bit easier than it actually is. With a little practice, however, you will become very good at it. Here are some useful tips for implementing time-out and making it work:

HOW LONG? The general rule of thumb is that a child should be in time-out one minute for every year of age. A two-year-old should be in time-out for two minutes, a three-year-old for three minutes, and so forth.

WHERE? One of the biggest problems for parents is finding a place to put their child for time-out. The best place is a time-out chair or naughty chair that is not an enjoyable place to be. This chair shouldn't be placed in front of the television or in a place where your child can play with toys. Don't put your child in her bedroom for time-out. There are too many fun things to do in there, and you don't want her associating the place where she sleeps with being punished. Having your child sit on the stairs is okay if your child will stay there. Some parents put their child in the bathroom. Bad idea. I have heard horror stories about children stuffing things down the toilet or causing the sink to overflow while in time-out. Many children have also locked themselves in the bathroom, either intentionally or by accident. Also, don't put your child anyplace where she can cause major destruction, such as next to the bookcase, where she can pull every book off the shelves. And don't put your child anywhere that is dangerous. For example, don't put her in the laundry room if there is a possibility that she can drink something poisonous. It is best to put your child in a chair someplace where you can keep an eye on her.

SET A TIMER. Another mistake that parents sometimes make is forgetting that their child is in time-out. Set a timer. This will remind you and also helps your child know when time-out is over. In addition, the timer, not the parent, indicates that time-out is over. When the bell goes off, the child knows that she can get up. It may even be best to use a digital timer, like the one on a microwave, so your child can see the time counting down.

PICK YOUR BATTLES. You will drive yourself crazy if you try to put your child in time-out for every single thing she does wrong. You cannot expect your child to be perfect. She can't be perfect— no one can. She doesn't know all the rules, and she can't follow every one of them all the time. So pick your battles and decide what is really important to you. Your list should include only a few major issues. Follow through on those and ignore the rest. What you will want to put on your list is any behavior that leads to your child being in danger, hurting herself or someone else, or destroying property. Once you choose bad behaviors that lead to time-out, be consistent in your efforts and always follow through.

STAYING IN TIME-OUT. One of the most difficult aspects of time-out is making your child stay. It is important that she stay there the entire time. Having a child struggle against time-out and then giving up and letting her go will defeat the entire purpose, and the next time you warn her that she will be put in time-out, she will not take you seriously. It will become an idle threat. But how do you keep your child there? It is easiest if your time-out is in a naughty chair. If she gets out, put her right back in. Be consistent and keep your cool. The calmer you are, the more likely that your child will be calm. If she sees you losing control, she will become more upset. If your child is persistent, there are two simple ways to keep her sitting. One way is to stand behind her and push down on her shoulders. You only need to do this when she tries to get up. When she is sitting calmly, you can keep your hands resting lightly on her shoulders. The other way to do it also involves standing behind her. Cross her arms over her chest and hold her hands lightly. She will not be able to stand up.

DON'T ENGAGE IN PROLONGED CONVERSATION. Many parents spend too much time explaining to their child why their behavior was wrong. Many children find this reinforcing, and they may misbehave to get your attention. So be careful about giving your child too much attention for doing something wrong by engaging in a prolonged conversation. It is better to tell your child in ten words or less: "You are going to time-out because you hit." After the time-out is over, feel free to talk to your child more about his misbehavior and what he can do better next time: "Next time, use your words." It can also be helpful to have your child explain to you why he was in time-out to make sure that he understands what he did wrong. You may be surprised sometimes by a child's interpretation of events. Rather than realizing he was in time-out for hitting his friend, he may think it's because he wasn't allowed to have his friend's toy.

DON'T LET TIME-OUT BE FUN. Children can have fun and make a game of almost anything. Time-out shouldn't be fun. Your child shouldn't be allowed to bring any toys with her into time-out. She shouldn't be allowed to watch television. One parent talked about having to take her child's shoes and socks off while in time-out because she would take them off, swing them around, and basically have fun. After a few times of losing her shoes and socks, she stopped playing and sat quietly.

MAINTAIN TIME-OUT IF SHE IS STILL SCREAMING AND CRYING. Don't let your child out of time-out if she is screaming and crying. Let your child out of time-out after the timer goes off but only if she is quiet. If she is screaming, inform her in a calm tone that she can get up when she is quiet. If you let her up while she is screaming, you will be reinforcing your child's screaming behavior. Don't reset the timer; just let her know that the moment she is quiet, she can get up. This doesn't mean that if she is quiet from the start she can get up right away. She has to wait for the timer to go off first.

YOUR CHILD STILL HAS TO FOLLOW DIRECTIONS. If you are putting your child in time-out because she didn't do something, such as putting away toys or getting dressed, make sure she does what you originally asked after the time-out is over. This will ensure that time-out is not being used as a means of escape. Otherwise your child may say to herself, "I don't want to put my toys away, so I'll just go into time-out for three minutes." Time-out should not be a way for your child to escape doing what she is told to do.

OTHER BASICS OF MANAGING BEHAVIOR

Be Consistent!

The key to changing behavior is being consistent. Once you decide to focus on a behavior that you want to change, you need to follow through each and every time. The reason for being consistent can be explained using two psychological terms: "consistent reinforcement" and "partial reinforcement." Consistent reinforcement involves getting something every time that you perform a certain behavior. Partial reinforcement is getting something only sometimes. Surprisingly, partial reinforcement makes bad behaviors persist much longer. Think of playing a slot machine. If you win every time you put a quarter in a slot machine, you will continue to play. Now imagine that you won five times in a row. On the sixth, seventh, and eighth try, however, nothing happened. You would realize that the machine has stopped paying out when you play. You would leave or at least move to another machine. Now think of the slot machine that has a partial-reinforcement schedule. The first time you get nothing. The second time you win two quarters. The third, fourth, and fifth time you win nothing. The seventh time you win seven quarters. The eighth time nothing. The ninth time twenty quarters. The tenth nothing. Are you going to keep playing? You sure are! This is because you hope and expect that if you keep persisting, you will win again. (And don't think that casinos don't understand these principles and use them! Unfortunately, in the long run you will lose money at the slot machines, but by using a partial-reinforcement schedule, they will have you playing for a longer time.)

The same principles are true for parenting. The parent who uses partial reinforcement, or partial punishment, is going to have a child who may be a behavioral problem. The child knows that his parent may or may not follow through. It is worth nagging or throwing a temper tantrum because it could pay off. The parent who uses consistent reinforcement, or consistent punishment, will have a child who is better behaved. In this case, the child knows the consequences for his behavior and knows that his parent is going to follow through. This doesn't mean that your child can never have a special unexpected treat or won't get away with something once in a while. It just lets everyone know what is expected and what will happen if misbehavior occurs.

The grocery store syndrome is an excellent example of the trap of partial reinforcement that parents fall into and why bad behavior often persists. Imagine the following scenario. It is one that we have all seen, and one that we all dread.

A mother is wheeling a grocery cart through a grocery store with her three-year-old seated in the front of the cart. She is hoping that she will be able to make it through the grocery store without mishap. She has a smile pasted on her face and is trying to engage her child in light banter, trying to distract him from all the junk food on the aisle shelves. She has successfully made it to the front of the grocery store and is now in the checkout line. Her child spots the candy bars near the cash register. (Do they put them there to torture parents?) He points to the M&Ms and asks for them. She says no. He points again. She says no. He starts whining. She says no. He starts crying. She says no. He starts crying as if his life depends on it. She says no. He starts screaming as if he were getting beaten. She looks around at everyone staring at her. She hands him the M&Ms. He smiles, wipes his eyes, and happily starts munching away.

What has happened in this scenario, and why is it so easy for us to imagine it and cringe? Everyone has seen this happen again and again, possibly with her own children. And it is likely that this same scene has happened with this same mother and child before. This is just another example of the powers of partial reinforcement. By giving in when he got really cranked up, the mother has just taught him to scream. The more persistent he is, the more likely it is that he is going to get that candy bar.

The same is true when it involves sleep. If you decide to put your child in his crib at bedtime and rescue him a half hour later because he is crying, you will simply teach him to cry. The next time he will cry even more. The message is to follow through and be consistent. Remember the issue of partial reinforcement, and remember that it leads to increased persistence of bad behavior.

The Soggy Potato Chip Theory

There is another theory that has been nicknamed the soggy potato chip theory. This theory states that a soggy potato chip is better than no potato chip at all. How does this relate to managing your child's behavior? Well, the corollary to this theory is that bad attention is better than no attention at all. To your child, attention from you is often the most important thing in her world. The best attention is obviously good attention (praise, spending time together, going for a walk), but the next best thing is bad attention. Bad attention is getting yelled at or being told not to do something. In your child's mind, if she has been playing quietly for the past hour and is being ignored, she may choose to misbehave. Why? Because staying quiet means that you will continue to ignore her, but spilling her juice is likely to get your attention. She may get scolded and have to clean it up, but it still will get your attention.

Rather than putting your child into this bind—"Would I rather get no attention or bad attention?"—do the opposite, which means that you should "catch 'em being good." That means paying attention to your child when she is being good. If she gets your attention for playing quietly, putting her toys away, or eating without spilling, there will be no reason for her to misbehave. If you respond to her positively for being good, she won't need to have you respond to her negatively for being bad.

Some parents respond to this advice by saying, "But when I pay attention to her when she is playing quietly, she inevitably acts up." Patricia noticed that this happened when her son, Joseph, was playing by himself with his toy cars. If she went in and talked to him about how well he was playing, he became aware of her presence and demanded that she play with him. If she didn't disturb him, he would continue to play quietly on his own, and she could get things done around the house. She had gotten to the point where she hated to disturb him because it would make him more demanding.

At first this may be a problem, with your child becoming more demanding of you. To deal with this, be calm and firm. Tell him you must do something else, but continue to praise him for being good. In time he will realize that your praise doesn't always mean you can stay and play. He will keep playing on his own, and the praise will reinforce his good behavior.

Reminders

- ✦ The key to changing behavior is being consistent.
- ✦ Focus on increasing good behavior and decreasing bad behavior.
- ✦ Reinforcement is the best way to get your child to do what you want.
- ✦ Provide acceptable choices.
- ✦ Don't ask questions when you intend to give commands.
- ✦ Make reasonable rules.

✦ Punishment is not a very effective way to change your child's behavior.

✦ Ignoring bad behavior and implementing time-out are excellent ways to stop your child from doing what you don't want.

✦ Sleep is similar to any other behavior; you can manage it just like any other behavior.

PART TWO

Establishing Good Sleep Habits

CHAPTER 4

"To Sleep, Perchance to Dream":
Getting Through the First Few Months

———

Joanne and Jim brought Daphne home when she was four days old. Joanne had had a cesarean section, so she stayed in the hospital a couple of extra days. Joanne was thrilled to finally be home. In the hospital Daphne had been an easygoing baby, seeming to cry less than the other babies in the nursery. The first few days at home went well. Joanne's mother helped during the day, and Jim helped at night. But then everything changed. Daphne got fussy. She seemed to cry all the time, and Joanne had no idea what to do. When Daphne wasn't crying, she was sleeping. Basically, Daphne spent 95 percent of the time she was awake crying. She slept for much of the afternoon, which was a relief to Joanne, but then she was up and crying from the moment Jim got home until everyone collapsed at midnight. At 2:30 in the morning it all started again, with Daphne up and crying. Joanne and Jim were frantic. Was being a parent always going to be like this?

———

The first days and weeks at home with a newborn can be overwhelming. All babies cry, and it always seems to be at the worst times, whether it is early evening when you are trying to make dinner or in the middle of the night. And although everyone claims that newborns sleep for up to twenty hours a day, no one seems to get any sleep. How can that be? Although your baby is sleeping many hours, it is only in thirty-minute to four-hour chunks of time. So your desire for an uninterrupted block of six to eight hours of sleep simply won't happen. In the meantime, try to get *some* sleep and remember: "This too will pass."

GETTING THROUGH THE FIRST SIX WEEKS

The first six weeks with a new baby can be extremely difficult. This is especially true with your first baby because everything is new and different, and you will have a great deal to learn about the day-to-day basics of taking care of a baby. It is also true with later children because you have to deal with balancing the needs of your newborn with the demands of your other children. It is all relative. Many parents with a firstborn are overwhelmed by the demands of a newborn. On the other hand, parents who have more than one child often comment on how they didn't realize how easy they had had it when they had only one child.

The difficulties of dealing with a newborn are compounded by parents' lack of sleep. Mothers often comment that the small amount of sleep they got during their last weeks of pregnancy, when they were waking on an hourly basis, seemed like heaven compared to the around-the-clock demands of a newborn. Also, sleep deprivation can contribute to postpartum depression.

The best thing you can do is nap when your baby naps, if possible. If the baby naps for an hour at 11:00 in the morning, you should too. Another idea is to hire a babysitter for your older child or children. Or you might treat your other children to a day away with their favorite person. And forget about returning all those phone calls from well-meaning friends and relatives. You should sleep. It will make you a happier person and a better parent. Consider screening your calls with an answering machine and discouraging drop-in visitors. Your friends and family will eventually have plenty of time with the baby. Also, make arrangements to get help.

Getting even a half-hour reprieve will make a large difference in your sanity.

While it is important simply to get through those first few weeks with a newborn, be sure to savor the moments. Babies grow so fast, and your baby will never be this small again. The time goes by quickly, and the next thing you know, your newborn has become a toddler and is no longer a tiny baby. As much as time may feel as if it is dragging during those first few weeks when you're pacing the floor with a crying newborn, you will realize later when you look back how fast the time really went.

DEALING WITH A NIGHT-OWL BABY

Some babies are night owls. They just don't seem to understand that they are supposed to be active during the day and sleep at night. In fact, during the day, things may seem easy. Your baby sleeps much of the time, wakes to feed, plays a little, and goes back to sleep. During the night, however, she seems to turn into a monster. She's awake and fussy, and nothing seems to calm her down.

What can you do? In the beginning, during the first week or two, not much. You may have to become a night owl yourself, knowing that eventually things will get better. Then, when your baby is one to three weeks old, there are some things that you can do to help get her clock on track. During the day, play with her as much as you can. Even if she seems to be sleeping soundly, wake her for feedings. Keep the shades open in her room and don't try to stay quiet all the time. Be your usual noisy daytime self. Don't turn the ringer off the phone or avoid turning on the dishwasher. This will also help ensure that your baby doesn't become the lightest sleeper in the world and force you to spend the next ten years of your life tiptoeing around the house when she is sleeping. During the night, play very little with her. Keep her room dark. Turn on only a night-light or low light for feedings and diaper changes. Be quiet and soothing. Move in slow motion. Eventually she will learn that daytime is for fun and night-time is for sleeping.

Maria's baby was a night owl. After coming home from the hospital, Miguel was fussy for the first four days. On the fifth day, Miguel slept much of the day, waking only three times for feedings. Each time he woke, Maria fed and changed him. Within ten minutes of being changed, he was back to sleep for three to four hours. Maria was elated, thinking that this was going to be easy. On the sixth day, though, she barely made it through her first sit-down dinner since having the baby before Miguel was awake and screaming. The next nine hours were a blur to Maria, with Miguel awake and fussy much of the time. At best, Miguel slept for twenty minutes at a time, and this pattern continued for the next nine days. Maria realized that she had to do something or she was going to lose her mind. The next day, Maria kept Miguel in a bassinet in the family room with her during the day. She turned the radio on and sang along with it. She brought Miguel into the kitchen when she prepared his bottle or got something to eat herself. Rather than putting him down right away after changing him, she held him and sang to him. She invited a friend over and encouraged her to hold and play with Miguel. That night, she put Miguel down in his crib in his room. She closed the shades and turned off the lights. When he awoke during the night, she kept him in his room and turned on only a low light. She kept her interactions with him to a minimum. After three days of keeping to this pattern, Miguel began to sleep longer at night and be more awake and alert during the day. Although he was still fussy at night, at least he would sleep for several hours at a time.

CRYING

Face it: babies cry. For them, crying is a way to communicate. It is their way of telling you when they are hungry, wet, need some cuddling, or just feel grumpy. Babies don't cry just "to exercise their lungs." They always cry for a reason.

On average, babies cry for three hours per day. That is a lot of crying. If your baby cries less than this amount, lucky you. If your baby cries more, think of her as a very communicative baby. It may help you to deal with the crying.

Babies Cry for Many Reasons

As you get to know your baby, you will begin to be able to determine what her cries mean. A whimpering cry may be her way of telling you that she is bored, whereas a scream implies that something hurts. Think of different cries as different words. Each cry can have a different meaning, or a certain cry may have many meanings. It is your job to try to figure out the possibilities, a task that will get easier over time as you get to know your baby.

The following are a few examples of why babies may cry.

PAIN. Obviously, babies cry when they are in pain. If nothing else works to soothe your baby, look for anything that may be causing pain. The strip method is helpful: strip your baby and look for anything that may be hurting. A common overlooked cause of pain is a hair that is wrapped around a finger, a toe, or some other delicate body part.

OVERSTIMULATION. Babies cry when they are overstimulated. You may have just been tickling and bouncing your baby. All of a sudden your baby goes from laughing along with you to crying. This may be the result of overstimulation. It just got to be too much for her. Loud noises, bright lights, or even too much hugging can all overcome a new baby. Having many visitors and being held by too many strangers can also be overstimulating.

BEING UNDRESSED. Some babies hate to be undressed. They start to cry and then howl as undressing progresses. It may not be because they are cold or you are inept at changing them. They just hate to be left with nothing close to their skin. The only remedy is to try to be fast when changing your child. Some find it helpful to put a cloth diaper or towel across the baby's stomach and chest when getting her undressed. This may be enough to calm her down.

BEING TOO COLD OR TOO HOT. Yes, either of these can make your baby cry. Babies often cry when they are first taken outdoors. It may not be the heat or chill per se but simply the change in temperature. A breeze can also upset a baby, no matter how perfect the temperature.

Ways to Respond to Crying

Here are just a few examples of things you can do to respond to your baby's cries.

FEED HER. Babies cry when they are hungry. If your baby hasn't eaten in a while, then try nursing her or giving her a bottle. If she just ate, you will need to try another strategy.

CHANGE HER. Babies also cry when they are wet or have a soiled diaper. One of the first things you can do when your baby cries is to check her diaper and change her if necessary.

SUCKING. Some babies simply want to suck, so try giving her a pacifier or encourage her to suck on her own fingers, and see if that calms her down. Don't always use a pacifier the minute your baby starts crying, but if you have tried everything else, a pacifier can be a real help.

HOLDING. Most babies love to be held. They are comforted by the physical contact. Don't worry about spoiling your baby by holding her too much. It is natural for your baby to want to be held. In many cultures babies are held all the time. They are strapped onto their mother's back or held by siblings or grandparents when parents aren't available. Studies have shown that babies who are held more than three hours a day cry much less. So invest in a quality front pack or sling and carry your baby around with you. It will be good for your baby and good for you, as your baby will be happy and content.

ROCKING. Some babies find gentle motion soothing, so try rocking her, pacing with her, or putting her in a swing. Some parents find a swing a lifesaver, whereas others find it of little help. Babies seem to either love or hate swings. If your baby is a swing lover, you are in luck.

VIBRATION. Other babies like the sensation of vibration. Take your baby for a car ride or get a vibrating infant seat.

MOVING. Just like adults, babies don't like to be in the same position or look at the same thing for too long. Unfortunately, unlike adults, they can't move themselves during those first few months. So if your baby has been in the same place for a while, try changing her position or moving her so that she can look at something new.

WARMTH. Babies often find warmth on their tummies to be soothing. Warm a receiving blanket carefully in a microwave or use a hot-water bottle. Touch the blanket or hot-water bottle to your cheek to make sure that it's not too hot.

SOOTHING NOISES. Soothing music, such as a classical piece, or the sound of a vacuum cleaner can calm a crying baby. Tapes that make the sound of a heartbeat can also be helpful.

SWADDLING. Many babies find swaddling to be very soothing. Also, swaddling can help your baby sleep, as babies often startle in their sleep. These naturally occurring jerks may jolt your baby awake. Swaddling will prevent these added awakenings.

VIDEOS. For some babies, putting on a video for fifteen minutes, such as the Baby Einstein series, can calm down even the fussiest little one. These developmentally appropriate videos are designed for newborns through toddlers and often captivate even the most upset baby.

A NEW PERSON. After an hour or even fifteen minutes, trying to deal with a screaming baby can get to the best of us. Your baby will sense your fatigue and frustration, which will simply make her more upset. Hand your baby over to someone else. This simple act may just do the trick.

DON'T WORRY. After spending time with your baby, you will begin to learn what your baby wants and what will make her more upset. There will also be times when you will be at your wits' end, when nothing you do seems to help your crying baby. Just remember that she is not crying for the sake of crying but because she is trying to tell you something. It is just as frustrating for her as it is for you.

COLIC

Colic is a problem that every parent has heard of and dreads. Colic is defined as excessive crying that occurs during the first three months of life in an otherwise healthy infant. Typically, a colicky infant cries two and a half times more than other infants. And the crying of a colicky infant is usually unrelenting and forceful. Colicky babies often draw their knees against their stomachs, flail their arms, and struggle when held. Anywhere from 10–25 percent of all newborns become colicky.

Most pediatricians use the rule of "threes" to diagnose colic. Babies who cry for three hours at a time, three days a week, for three weeks are termed colicky. Surprisingly, this may not be all that different from normal fussy crying. Remember, the average baby will cry for about three hours a day at six weeks of age, which is a lot of crying. What differentiates a baby with colic, though, is that the crying occurs all at once. Other babies may cry for a total of three hours per day, but it occurs in short spurts throughout the day.

Colic, which is usually not diagnosed until at least three weeks of age, peaks at six weeks of age. Then, around three months, babies with colic will seem miraculously cured.

Until he was nineteen days old, Calvin was the "perfect baby." He would cry, sleep, and eat, all in fairly predictable ways. His parents thought that he was the best baby ever—that is, until day nineteen, which started like any other day. Calvin woke twice during the early morning to feed. Then throughout the day he woke to feed, spent some time awake in his swing, and cried when he was hungry or needed to be changed. At 4:00 in the afternoon, everything changed. Calvin started screaming. He couldn't be calmed. His mother gave him a bottle, she changed him, she rocked him, she tried distracting him with his favorite toy, and she paced. She even called the pediatrician because Calvin's behavior was so unusual. By the time her husband came home at 6:00, she was frantic. They took Calvin for a drive in the car. They turned on the vacuum cleaner. They did everything humanly possible. Nothing worked. Calvin finally fell asleep from exhaustion at 8:30, after screaming uncontrollably for four and a half straight hours. Life continued this way for weeks. Calvin would be fine all day until, as his parents described it, the "witching hour struck." Without fail, Calvin would start screaming uncontrollably at about 4:00 each day.

No one is certain what causes colic. The word "colic" comes from the Greek word *kolikos*, the adjective of *kolon*, which means the large intestine. This term relates to the belief that colic is caused by some type of abdominal or intestinal pain. The cause of colic is unclear and may be different for individual babies. Most people claim that colic is caused by excessive gas. And most babies with colic seem to be gassy, though whether the gas is causing the colic or whether the incessant crying is causing the gas is not clear. Other causes have also been proposed, although there is little support for any of them. Some say colic is related to a milk allergy (very rare), an immature gastrointestinal tract (why then does it occur in some babies and not all?), overfeeding or underfeeding (unlikely), inappropriate handling of the infant by the parent (but colic occurs equally in first, second, and even fifth babies, so experience has nothing to do with it), or heredity (it does not run in families). Or, as is most likely, there is no real cause. The excessive crying is just an extreme variation of normal. If the average baby cries almost three hours a day, that means there are some babies who cry for only one hour and others who predictably cry for six hours.

Colic not only involves lots of crying but also can disrupt sleep. Babies with colic sleep less during the night and wake more frequently—not exactly what you need after dealing with a crying baby all day. Colicky babies are also more restless when they sleep. Their sleep is more disrupted, and they awaken more easily. During the day it is harder to predict when they will nap and for how long. So not only are parents of babies with colic sleep deprived, but it is much more difficult for them to get other things done when the baby is sleeping because it is so hard to predict their baby's behavior.

Along with not knowing the cause of colic, there is no known cure or treatment. But parents will try everything. They change their baby's diet. They change their own diet if the mother is breast-feeding (such as eliminating caffeine, chocolate, or milk products). They change the temperature of the formula if they are bottle-feeding. Some doctors prescribe medications or suggest rhythmic movement, such as riding in a moving car or being placed in a moving swing. Try everything! Your attempts may not work or may work only some of the time, but doing nothing can be even more stressful.

The most important person to treat during colic is yourself. Try to get through it while maintaining your sanity. To do so, you need help. You need to get away from the situation. Take a walk. Take a break. Beg every friend you have to watch the baby for a half hour. Put on headphones.

Unfortunately, even after the colic has resolved, sleep problems may continue. Babies whose sleep is not regular often continue to have disrupted sleep. The reasons for this are many. Babies who do not consolidate their sleep during the period of colic may become used to waking frequently. Because of the colic, these babies are less likely to have strategies to soothe themselves back to sleep and can be more likely to require parental attention to return to sleep. Also, it can be hard to distinguish between your baby's continuing to have colic or simply having a sleep problem. One way to decide is to observe whether your baby has gotten over the incessant daytime crying. If she seems fine during the day, then it is likely that colic has also resolved at night.

SLEEP AND BREAST-FEEDING

One of the surprises of parenting that may fall in the category of "no one ever told me" is that breast-fed babies typically sleep for shorter periods and are usually older when they finally begin to sleep through the night.

Why do breast-fed babies sleep for shorter periods? Since breast milk is much easier for babies to digest than formula, it means shorter intervals between feedings. So a baby at eight weeks may still be breast-feeding every two or three hours throughout the night, while a bottle-fed baby may be sleeping for up to four to six hours a night. These trends don't hold for all babies, of course. Your baby may do the exact opposite. But as a whole, these are the likely effects of breast-feeding and bottle-feeding on your baby's sleeping pattern.

Breast-fed babies are also more likely to fall asleep while feeding and thus develop a sleep association with nursing. This means that when they wake during the night, they need to be nursed back to sleep. It is also more difficult to break this habit because the mother is so closely associated with breast-feeding. During the night the mother may have a reflexive letdown of her milk when she sees the baby. She smells like milk. It is hard to tell a baby that nursing is not allowed when he smells the milk (see Chapter 10 for suggestions on how to deal with these issues).

There is no question, though, that a breast-fed baby can be a champion sleeper. The most important thing is to avoid falling into the trap of nursing your baby to sleep (although it is quite tempting). Instead, nurse your baby earlier in the bedtime routine. Change him into pajamas after nursing. Or nurse somewhere else in the house and then head to the bedroom for some cuddle time in the rocking chair before putting your baby to bed (or have Dad or another person do this part). Does this mean that you can never nurse your baby to sleep? Of course not. There are times when you will nurse your baby to sleep, especially when he is sick or extra fussy. However, you want it to be an exception rather than the norm.

As a nursing mom myself (my daughter nursed until twenty months), I can attest to the importance of separating breast-feeding from sleep. I exclusively breast-fed for six months but always put her down awake at bedtime and for naps. My daughter was a great sleeper, with the usual bumps along the way such as when she was ill or when she decided that pulling up to standing was much more fun than sleeping.

SOOTHING STRATEGIES

One thing that you can do during your child's early months is help him learn to soothe himself. This will make going to sleep much easier in later months. Most babies are very good at soothing themselves. It will just take some minor effort on your part to encourage this activity. And it is important to realize that there is a fine balance between responding to your child's needs and giving him the chance to soothe himself. Both are important. It is just a matter of figuring out when to intervene and when to let him be. You don't want to ignore your child's needs, but you also don't want to smother him and prevent him from developing ways to soothe himself.

Here are some suggestions to help your baby learn to soothe himself.

SUCKING. Some babies find sucking on their thumb, fingers, fist, or wrist soothing. When your baby is crying, try gently placing his hand in his mouth to see if it will calm him. If you do not want to encourage your child to suck his thumb, then try another strategy.

ZONING OUT. Many times we try to distract a crying baby with a toy or by making faces. If you do this and your child turns away or closes his eyes, take this as a message that he needs to zone out. Let him. He may need some peace and quiet. Take the toys away and let him stare at the wall or a spot on the ceiling.

FAVORITE POSITION. Some babies have a favorite position, such as on their back, on their side, or scrunched up against the side of the crib. Once you figure out your baby's favorite position, put him in that position when he is upset and see if it helps him calm down. Once he falls asleep, be sure to shift him to his back, to decrease the risk of SIDS. And, as mentioned earlier, some babies are calmed by being swaddled, whereas others hate being confined.

LEAVE HIM ALONE. If your baby pushes you away or turns from you, he is giving you the message to leave him alone. Don't take this personally. Rather, take this as a positive sign that your baby can calm himself. Turn him away from you so that he can see something else or put him down on a blanket on the floor.

LESS NOISE, PLEASE. Some babies simply enjoy quiet. Try turning off the music or the television. Get him away from brothers and sisters who are playing loudly. Imagine yourself in a restaurant or a store where the noise is too loud, making you feel edgy. Your baby can feel that way at times also. This is not to say that you should always be quiet around your baby, but if he is fussy, try toning it down a bit.

SIX WEEKS TO THREE MONTHS

Your baby is now six weeks old, no longer a newborn. It is time to start thinking about establishing good sleep habits. By starting early, you will help your baby sleep through the night at a very young age and you will prevent future sleep problems.

Establish Good Sleep Habits Early

Between the ages of six weeks and three months is the best time to establish good sleep habits. If this is your second child, you know how crucial it is to start your baby off right and prevent future problems. It is so much easier now than to have to do sleep training when your baby is six months, a year, or even two years old. Physiologically your baby is at the point when she is able to sleep for prolonged stretches of time. This is also one of the easiest times to encourage good sleep habits because your baby can't get too far. She can't climb out of her crib yet, and she has not moved to a bed. Developmental milestones that can interfere with sleep, such as rolling over and separation anxiety, also haven't developed. And you are probably at the point where you are ready to get more than four continuous hours of sleep.

There are three key things that you can do now to help your baby start sleeping for longer stretches.

SLEEP SCHEDULE. Start establishing a sleep schedule. This schedule should include a set bedtime, a set wake time, and set naptimes (either following the clock or using the two-hour rule; see Chapter 7). A consistent feeding schedule will also help set a more general daily routine.

SLEEP ROUTINES. Even at this young age, your baby will benefit from a bedtime routine and a naptime routine. At this age, it may be as simple as a sponge bath, diaper change, pajamas and a lullaby at bedtime, and just a diaper change and lullaby at naptimes. Your bedtime routine may take only five minutes, but it will signal to your baby that it is sleep time.

PUT DOWN DROWSY BUT AWAKE. The most important aspect of getting a baby to sleep through the night (see Chapter 6 for more details) is to have your baby learn to soothe herself to sleep. Babies need to be able to put themselves to sleep without your intervention. The reason is that all babies, as well as all adults, wake during the night. This is normal. What is problematic is not the nighttime wakings but the inability to return to sleep. Your baby needs to learn to soothe herself to sleep so that when she wakes for a moment in the middle of the night, she can immediately put herself back to sleep.

Sometime between six and twelve weeks, start putting your baby down when she is still awake. She doesn't have to be wide-awake; she can be groggy, but she can't be sound asleep. Put her down in her crib or wherever you intend for her to sleep all night. Give her something to look at. Some parents have found it helpful to save a favorite toy to engage their baby at sleep times. The favorite toy can be almost anything.

Beverly found that her son Jason loved looking at a funny-looking stuffed animal that a friend gave them. It resembled a bug and a frog at the same time. Whatever it was, Jason loved to stare at it. This froglike bug helped Jason make the transition into sleep. Beverly would put Jason and the toy in the crib. For a few moments Jason would fuss, until he spotted the animal. Then he would just stare at it, and within a few moments he would start to zone out, eventually sucking on his fingers and falling asleep. Once Jason was able to fall asleep on his own at such a young age, he continued to be a great sleeper. Many other parents were in awe of Jason, who would go to bed at 8:00 at night, not to be heard from again until 7:00 the next morning.

The key to getting Jason and all babies to sleep through the night from an early age is to put them down awake!

Another choice to help make the transition into sleep easier is to hang a mirror on the side of your baby's crib so that he can look at himself. A mobile will also work, although it may not be best for you to turn it on so that it spins or plays music, since your baby then will want it turned on in the middle of the night when he awakens. It may seem like nothing to get up, turn the mobile on, and go back to sleep, especially in comparison with being up with your baby for an hour, but this will eventually get old, and you will appreciate longer stretches of unbroken sleep. So if you believe that you are setting your baby up for another bad habit, try to come up with another option.

Begin putting your baby down when he is still awake at bedtime and also at naptimes. The more practice that your baby gets putting himself to sleep, the quicker the process works. He will fall asleep on his own, and you will get the sleep that you need. Remember, however, that breast-fed babies are notorious for taking longer to fall asleep on their own and to sleep through the night. You can begin the process early, but you may not want to start until your baby is eight to ten weeks old. Don't wait too long, though. The earlier the better. Remember, once your baby gets older—that is, at least five months—the process of getting your child on a sleep schedule and to sleep through the night gets more difficult.

When you start putting your baby down awake at this age, consider these times as practice sessions. Babies this young should not be left to cry for a prolonged period. Instead, make it a practice session and see if it works. Put him down, say, "Night-night," leave, and see what happens. If your baby starts to whimper and fuss, wait a few minutes. He may surprise you by settling down and falling asleep. If he starts to get very upset, go and get him and do whatever you normally do to help him fall asleep. Wait until the next sleep time or wait for another day and try again. Often parents are stunned by their baby's self-soothing abilities. Whereas they thought their baby had to be rocked or nursed to sleep, it may not be true at all. Many babies are happy to be put down, look at their favorite toy, and drift off to slumberland on their own.

Scheduled Nighttime Feedings

Around this age, try adding a scheduled feeding around 10:30 to 11:30 at night. Some refer to this as a "focal feeding" or a "dream feeding." It feels terrible to parents to drift happily off to sleep at 11:00 at night, only to have their baby wake them thirty minutes later. So wake your baby before you go to bed and feed her. You'll be surprised at how well this works. She'll likely barely wake up, but will happily eat. Both of you can then sleep soundly for three to four hours before the next feeding.

Ron started doing a dream feeding with his daughter when she was six weeks old. His wife went to bed at 10:00 and he would wake the baby around 11:00. These dream feedings became his favorite part of the day, as they would cuddle in the rocking chair in the baby's room while it felt like the rest of the world was sleeping. He continued doing these feedings every night until she was almost eight months old. She didn't need the feeding any longer, but he hated to give up this special time.

Daytime Feedings

Making changes in your child's daytime feeding schedule may also help your child sleep longer at night. You can try moving your baby's feedings closer together during the day to fit in an extra feeding. This can help your baby get the nutrition he needs during the day, making nighttime feedings less necessary. Flavia did this with four-month-old Gabrielle. Gabrielle usually had a bottle every three and one-half hours. When Flavia switched Gabrielle to a bottle every three hours, she was able to fit in five feedings during the day, rather than four. Gabrielle consequently dropped one of her nighttime feedings, only getting up once at night rather than twice.

For other babies, who can't seem to go more than an hour or two between feedings, you may need to gradually lengthen the time between feedings to help them sleep longer.

Walk, Don't Run

During the night, when you hear your baby begin to stir, walk, don't run to him. You will be surprised how often he'll fall back to sleep on his own. Remember, all babies naturally wake up throughout the night. Your baby may simply be stirring, ready to return right back to sleep. By going to him too quickly, you may actually be waking him up.

Susanne found this to be the case with her daughter Savannah. When Savannah woke up at night, Susanne would always make a quick trip to the bathroom and feed the cat so the cat wouldn't howl before going in to nurse her. Half the time, Savannah had fallen back to sleep in the three minutes it took Susanne to get to her room.

Transitioning to a Crib

In the first few weeks to months, many parents have their babies sleep in a bassinet, infant seat, or other smaller space. The crib often seems too huge for such a tiny baby, and a bassinet can easily be set up in the parents' bedroom. If you plan to have your baby eventually sleep in a crib, you need to make the transition by three months. Wait much longer than three months, and it will be much more difficult for your baby. After three months, habits are set and the change in sleeping location will feel too new and different. When you start the transition, you can do it all at once or gradually. For a gradual change, start with just naps or just bedtime in the crib. Once your baby is used to the new location, move on to napping and sleeping in the crib all night. Some babies do much better in the crib if you put them down in a corner of the crib, rather than in the middle. Having one of their sides and their head up against the crib bumpers may help them feel more secure. Putting rolled-up receiving blankets on all sides of your baby will also do the trick.

Linda found that when she put her three-month-old son Jack into his crib, he would cry and wake up every hour throughout the night. When he slept in his car seat, though, he would fall asleep quickly and sleep for up to six hours straight. So she went for a gradual change. First, she literally put the car seat in the crib at bedtime, making sure that it couldn't topple over and that Jack couldn't reach anything. After a week, she started putting Jack in his crib just at bedtime, moving him to his car seat when he woke up an hour later. Jack started sleeping longer and longer in his crib without waking up, and about a week later Linda no longer needed to move him to his car seat during the night.

Reminders ————————————————————————

- ✦ The first six weeks with a newborn can be difficult. Get sleep whenever you can.
- ✦ Babies cry, and they cry for many reasons. Crying is a baby's way of communicating. Learn what your baby's cries mean and how to respond to your crying baby's needs.

✦ Coping with a baby with colic is difficult, but it is manageable.

✦ Between the ages of six weeks and three months is the best time to establish good sleep habits that will help your baby sleep through the night and prevent future sleep problems.

CHAPTER 5

Bedrooms, Bedtimes, and Bedtime Routines

"Each night around 8:00, while Zachary is quietly playing, I begin to dread the ordeal of bedtime. By 9:30, Zachary is overtired, and it becomes impossible to get him to bed without a fight. By the time he is finally asleep, it is 10:30, and I am tense and exhausted. This is not the life I envisioned."

SET BEDTIMES

As mentioned previously, one of the more important things that you can do for your baby (after proper nutrition and lots of love, of course) is setting a bedtime. Every night your baby should be going to bed at about the same time. A typical baby bedtime is between 7:00 and 8:30 at night. Your baby won't be going to bed this early, though, until between three and five months of age.

Keeping your baby up past 8:30 may not be a good idea. Babies need sleep—and lots of it. However, many parents keep their baby up longer than they should. In fact, if you have to struggle to get your baby to sleep, you may be more likely to keep your baby up later. This may be because you can't bear to face the "sleep showdown" or because you think that if you wait until your baby is very tired, he will go to sleep more easily and quickly. Unfortunately, just the opposite happens. The more tired a baby becomes, the more wired he will be, and the more wired he is, the harder time he will have falling asleep. Many a parent of a toddler has commented, "See, he's not tired. It is ten o'clock at night, and he is running around the living room like a banshee." Actually, that is a sign that he is extremely tired. Studies show that young children often become more active the more tired they are. So don't put off your baby's bedtime!

One reason some babies go to bed so late is that working parents feel that evenings are the only time they have to spend with their child. Debbie, the mother of two-year-old Kevin, kept Kevin until 10:00 p.m. Her husband, Tony, rarely got home before 8:00 at night, and she said that if they didn't keep Kevin up late, Tony would never get to see his child. Although this may seem like a good decision for the sake of the parent-child relationship, it is not a good idea to sacrifice your child's sleep. Babies' sleep is very important to their development. Instead, try to rearrange schedules so that time together can occur but your child can still get to bed on time.

Having a set bedtime routine helps to set your baby's internal clock. As adults, we have external cues to keep our internal clocks on track. We look at the clock, we eat meals at the same time, we go to work at the same time, and we watch television shows that are shown at specific times. These cues help to make us tired at our usual bedtime, and most people have no problem falling asleep. Since babies cannot tell time, they need us to set their internal time clocks throughout the day by their daily activities. They need to eat meals at basically the same time every day, and they need to go to bed at about the same time. By keeping your child's internal clock always consistent, she will fall asleep more easily and quickly.

Having a set bedtime is also good because it helps parents know when to start the bedtime routine and reduces the chance that they will procrastinate getting the baby to sleep. Sometimes when your two-and-a-half-year-old is playing quietly at 7:30 p.m.—perhaps for the first time all day—it is hard to get up the nerve to announce that it is bedtime and start the ensuing battle. But putting it off will only make the entire process harder. Then everyone is tired and tempers are short, including yours.

Finally, it is important for parents to have time to themselves at night. To be a good parent, you need time to yourself, whether to connect with your spouse, enjoy a show on television, or catch up with friends or family.

ROUTINES

Babies and children love routines and relish schedules. They like to know what is going to happen next. They are also better behaved when things follow a known pattern. Routines provide your child with a sense of security, and they enable your child to have a sense of control in a world governed by adult demands. Routines also give a framework in which to learn new skills. In the early weeks, you will need to follow your child's schedule, but by three months, provide increasing structure to your baby's day. Have consistent mealtimes, playtimes, and sleep times. As you can imagine, if the times of other activities are constantly changing, sleep patterns will also be irregular. Remember, though, that during that first year, just when you think you have established some predictability, things will change. That is okay. A routine in place for even a few days will help tremendously.

Routines help parents, too. They provide a sense of control and an expectation of what is going to happen in a particular day. You will know what time your child will have meals and when he will sleep. Knowing that you are going to get some free time during your child's 1:00 naptime will help you keep your patience during a morning when you can't get anything done. Routines also end arguments over what is going to happen next. If your children always watch a video after dinner, then there is no discussion of whether you will play outside with them when you need to wash the dishes and clean up the kitchen.

You should allow your child to help establish daily routines by incorporating something your child does naturally into his daily routine.

Sophie, sixteen months, likes to put her cup in the sink after every meal. Her mother, Jennifer, encourages Sophie to do this. This daily routine helps Sophie to understand that mealtime is over and it is time to go on and do something else.

Sam, age three, goes around and says good night to the family pets before going up to bed. It can take a while to find the family's dog and three cats, but the routine helps Sam make the transition to bedtime.

If your household is chaotic, start by adding routines to the beginning and end of the day. Start with morning time or bedtime. Make a list of what needs to get done, figure out a good order, and start there. Be realistic. Trying to cram too much into too little time will only frustrate you and your child. For example, getting dressed and eating breakfast can take a toddler twice as long as you would like. Rather than rushing her, provide more time so that mornings can be relaxing without constant reminders to hurry up. The same is true in the evenings, before bedtime. Use reminders to let your child know what is going to happen next. "After you brush your teeth, we'll read a bedtime story" or "After this last story, we'll go kiss Mommy good night." As you get mornings and evenings under control, start adding routines throughout the day. Have meals at the same time each day. Schedule set naptimes and playtimes. Your day doesn't have to be regimented, but with certain specific markers of things happening throughout the day, your entire day will go more smoothly, and both you and your child will be happier.

BEDTIME ROUTINES

Bedtime routines help your baby become sleepy and prepare him to sleep through the night. Beginning these practices at a very young age, even by six to eight weeks, will help your baby sleep and can prevent sleep problems later in life. Your bedtime routine with your baby can be just about anything that you want. There are basically only two essential factors that need to be incorporated. One is making the end of the routine calm. The other important component is having the last part of the routine occur in your child's bedroom. Many families use the child's bedroom only as a place to go when it is time to sleep. For the child, this practice can make the bedroom seem like a place of banishment. So be sure to spend at least the last ten minutes of your child's bedtime routine in his bedroom. This will help him associate his bedroom with good feelings, a place where cuddling occurs and quality time is spent.

Bedtime routines help make sleep times and wake times significantly different and distinguishable for your child. There are many things you can integrate into your bedtime routine. Putting on special types of clothes, namely pajamas, and having certain rituals, such as taking a bath or brushing teeth, help your child learn the distinction between daytime and nighttime.

If your child hates baths or finds them too stimulating, do the bath earlier in the day. Brushing teeth is always a good habit to start young (be sure to ask your pediatrician about how to brush new baby teeth). Read or make up a story, say silly rhymes, sing a song, play a favorite quiet game, imagine nice dreams, or say prayers. Sing the ABC song or count to twenty. Talk quietly about what you did today and what you are going to do tomorrow. With older children, discuss any worries or concerns. Talk about what the best thing was that happened that day, and what the worst was. Cross off the day on the calendar. Cuddle.

Whatever your routine is, make it yours, make it special, and make it consistent. Starting young with a bedtime routine helps start a tradition that will continue throughout your child's growing years. Everyone will know that this is a special time and that it involves good-quality one-on-one time. It also helps establish a safe space for your child to tell you what is happening in his life.

Below are some of the most important tips related to bedtime routines.

+ **Consistency, consistency, consistency.** Be sure that it is the same every day. For example, Sharon always followed what she referred to as the *"Rule of the Four Bs"*: bath, breast (well, actually, she called it "boob"), book, and bed. Your child will be more relaxed if she knows what is coming next. The more relaxed she is, the more likely she will go to bed easily and fall asleep quickly. Compare these two routines for these two different children:

Stacey

> DAY 1. Bath, pajamas, teeth, story
> DAY 2. Story, bath, teeth, pajamas
> DAY 3. Story, pajamas, teeth, kiss good night
> DAY 4. Pajamas, teeth, song, drink of water

Rebecca

> DAY 1. Bath, pajamas, story, kiss good night
> DAY 2. Bath, pajamas, story, kiss good night
> DAY 3. Bath, pajamas, story, kiss good night
> DAY 4. Bath, pajamas, story, kiss good night

Clearly, you would expect that Rebecca would go to bed more easily because her bedtime routine is predictable. She knows what to expect. Not only is Rebecca's routine the same every night, but she is also read a familiar story at bedtime. A fa-

vorite story is often better than a new story every night because it is relaxing. Save new stories for daytime hours.

+ **Start early.** You can begin to establish your baby's bedtime routine right from the start. In the beginning, your
routine may be only five or ten minutes long and include
just a sponge bath and a song. As your baby gets older,
your routine will grow with her.

+ **Head in one direction.** Make sure your bedtime routine is
always heading in the same direction. Once you are upstairs, head straight to your child's room for pajamas and
books. You don't want a routine that moves all over the
place, such as bath upstairs, then downstairs for snack,
then back upstairs to read books on your bed, and then finally to bed in your child's room. Simplify it—instead,
make it snack downstairs, bath upstairs, and stories and
hugs in your child's room.

+ **Keep it short and sweet . . .** Keep your bedtime routine
short and sweet. A bedtime routine is anywhere from
twenty to forty-five minutes (if it includes a bath). Taking two hours to get ready for bed is not a bedtime routine, it's an evening activity!

+ **. . . but include everything.** Don't make the routine
overly long or involved, but be sure to include in your
routine everything that is important and necessary. If
your child is toilet trained, then make sure that going
to the bathroom is part of the routine. Get that last drink
of water before saying good night. Make sure that
everyone has gotten hugs and kisses, so there aren't
any late-night calls for a hug from Daddy or a good
night to the dog. If everything is included, then you
will know that any requests from your child later on are
not necessary ones, and you will feel better about ignoring them.

✦ **Don't include anything scary.** Don't play monsters or tell scary stories right before bed. If you do, no wonder your toddler is afraid to be alone in the dark and is having nightmares.

✦ **Make the last activity the favorite one.** The last thing in your child's routine should be her favorite. So save snuggle time, reading a story, or playing with a special game or toy for last to encourage your child to head to bed.

✦ **Bedtime chart.** For an older child, a bedtime chart can make things much easier. Either draw or cut out pictures that show all the steps in your bedtime routine and paste them on a chart in order, such as a picture of a bathtub, then pajamas, and then two storybooks. Your child will enjoy following along with the chart, and it will keep everyone on track ("Nope, only two bedtime books; that's what the chart says").

Every family has its own bedtime routines and rituals, and these may change as the child gets older. It will take some time to develop your own particular routine that is enjoyable and relaxing for everyone.

Steven works all day, often leaving in the morning before his children are even awake. For him, bedtime is his wind-down time with his two children, John, age four, and Karen, fifteen months. Due to his work he often misses the children's dinnertime but tries to make sure that he is always home for their bedtime. While his wife gives one child a bath, Steven spends some time talking and playing with the other. John loves to build things, so every night Steven helps him build a "bigger and better" tower. While building, they often talk about what happened that day, and simply connect.

Karen is a cuddler. Steven usually spends lots of cuddle time with Karen and reads to her from her favorite book, Goodnight Moon. *When both children are in their pajamas, he sings silly songs to both of them. Then comes a kiss, a hug, and "Eskimo kisses" for everyone.*

At one and a half, Joey knows that the last thing before bedtime is saying ABCs and counting to ten. Joey's mother points to each letter and number on a wall hanging as she says them. Joey always looks forward to this and often asks his mother to do it again. Following the ABCs and counting, last hugs and kisses are given, and Joey goes down in his crib.

Once all teeth are brushed and pajamas are on, Susan reads to her twins, Ryan and Alex, age two. She always reads poems from Where the Sidewalk Ends. *She tries to read at least one new one every night, but Ryan and Alex always insist on hearing their favorites night after night. After all poems are read, Susan sings "Puff the Magic Dragon" to them while cuddling on the overstuffed chair in their bedroom. Susan has been singing this song to them every night at bedtime since they were infants.*

On days when you don't have time for the entire bedtime routine, do an abbreviated one. Sing only one song or read only one poem rather than several. If you don't do any part of the routine, though, you may pay for it because it may take your child twice as long to settle down. For some, though, not doing the entire bedtime routine will backfire, as you end up arguing about only reading one book instead of two. This may end up taking the same amount of time as doing the full routine, so things may go much more smoothly if you just do the entire routine.

THE BEDTIME TRANSITION

Many a parent has heard the bedtime plea of "Just five more min-utes" or "I don't wanna!" Going to bed can be difficult for children. It signifies the end of a day, which is especially hard when it has been an exciting day, such as a holiday or a birthday. Many children also hate to miss anything. They may feel that all of the fun starts after they have gone to bed. Little do they know that much of what is happening is bill paying and doing the dishes. Another reason that your child may resist going to bed is that she has a hard time with transitions.

To help alleviate bedtime resistance, there are several things that have been found to be helpful. For one, help make the transi-tion easier for your child. Warn her. Five to ten minutes before bedtime should begin, let her know that bedtime is coming. That way she can finish the puzzle she is working on or stop the video at an appropriate place. By the time your child is eighteen months, this tactic will be helpful. Starting at such a young age will also help her begin to understand the concept of time. Some parents find it helpful to set a timer at the five-minute mark. This helps al-leviate the pressure on the parent: "Hey, the timer says it is time to go to bed." This can carry you for a long time before your child realizes that you are the one who set the timer.

Bedtime routines are also a great way to deal with the bedtime resister, especially if the bedtime routine includes something that your child loves to do, such as reading a favorite story. Bedtime rou-tines give your child the time she needs to make the transition to going to bed.

How do you deal with a dawdler? One way to deal with this problem is to extend the time you allot to getting ready for bed. This is supposed to be a calm, soothing time, not a mad rush. Hurrying your child may just make her resist more and get her so worked up that she will have a hard time settling down to fall asleep. If you know that your daughter takes twenty minutes rather than ten to get up the stairs and into her pajamas, start earlier and give her twenty minutes to get it done. This way you won't get frustrated by her being a slowpoke. Remember that she can't tell time, so if you start her bedtime routine at 7:00 rather than 7:30, she won't know the difference (unless she has a favorite TV show that comes on at 7:00—though you can always decide to tape it).

Make getting ready for bed into a game. Play "beat the clock." Set a timer for a reasonable amount of time. If your child is ready before the timer goes off, she gets an extra story or a special treat. Have your child choose how she is going to go to bed. Is she going to walk backward, skip, tiptoe like a mouse, or stomp like a monster? Playing such a game gives your child some control over bedtime and makes going to bed more fun.

Another idea is to use incentives. Make the last part of the bedtime routine the most enjoyable part. Don't wait to brush teeth until after stories, do it before. Sing your child's favorite song last. Allow time for some playtime after putting on pajamas. Dan found that once he switched the order of his three-year-old son's bedtime routine so that they played together with his G.I. Joes in his room once everything else was done, getting ready for bed went much more smoothly and there was no more stalling.

TRANSITIONAL OBJECTS

Many babies make the transition to sleep more easily if they have a favorite object with them. These are called transitional objects. Some parents call them "loveys." The object can be just about anything. For most children it is something soft and cuddly, like a teddy bear or blanket. Amy, age three, took Bunny with her everywhere. Bunny went to the store, on car rides, and especially to bed for naptimes and bedtime. Soft and cuddly isn't the rule for all loveys. Calvin's favorite thing in the world was a small hammer that he had found in his father's toolbox. Calvin wouldn't go anywhere without it, especially to bed. Recent studies show that about 60 percent of young children have a lovey by the end of their first year, although, interestingly, the specific lovey often changes over time, with a different object being a favorite at different times. A lovey can be important, as it can help a child bridge the gap between complete dependence on parents and independence, and provides a stable and steady comforting presence. A lovey can go anywhere and be anywhere when other security objects, namely Mom and Dad, may not be there. So a lovey can go to Grandma's house for the afternoon, will be there when a favorite parent is at the store, and, in terms of sleep, is there all night.

Helping Your Child Develop an Attachment

Some children never have an attachment object. This is fine and doesn't mean anything about your child in general. However, you can try and help your child become attached to something. Find an object that your child seems to prefer, such as a cuddly stuffed animal or a blanket. Every time you hold and feed your child, such as while nursing or giving a bottle, have your child hold the object. When your child needs comforting, such as after falling down or when he meets a new person, hand him the object. Danielle did this to help her son, Stefan, make the transition from twirling her hair to soothe himself. His endless twirling of her hair at bedtime and every time he got upset was making it impossible for her to leave him with his father or a babysitter. In addition, it hurt! For two weeks, she would let him twirl her hair but also gave him a stuffed bunny to hold while he did so. At the end of the two weeks, she began gently removing his hand from her hair and handing him the bunny. After a few weeks, she knew that the transition was successful when Stefan immediately sought out his bunny when a stranger came to visit.

Losing a Lovey

One of the saddest things for a child is losing a lovey. This has happened to many a child. Favorite things often get left at the grocery store or on vacation, or just disappear to the same mysterious place matching socks seem to go. If this happens to your child, you are going to have to deal with it. Don't pretend it hasn't happened. Don't pretend that it's no big deal. It's very hurtful to a child to tell him that he's a big boy now and doesn't need his lovey or that he's too old for a teddy anyway. He may not wish to be a big boy right then, and this has little to do with how old he is. Some children will allow a replacement, but don't be surprised if your child doesn't take to another object.

Get a Duplicate!

If your child has one incredibly special lovey and doesn't change objects from month to month, do whatever you can to have another on hand. If your child finds a love object, buy two or three if you can. Have a spare in case the original gets lost or misplaced, or is just in the wash. Katarina found a matching fuzzy blanket to her daughter Katelyn's favorite blanket. She would rotate them each week. One would go in the wash and the other would go in her crib. This way, both blankets were equally loved in case one got lost.

Transitional Objects and Sleep

Some studies have shown that incorporating a transitional object into your baby's bedtime can help your baby go to sleep on her own and sleep through the night. One study found that something reminiscent of Mom did the trick. In this study mothers wore a T-shirt all day. At night they put the T-shirt in the crib with their baby. Amazingly, it worked. The smell of the baby's mother on the T-shirt calmed the babies and helped them fall asleep. (Note: If you try this, tie the T-shirt in a knot for safety reasons.)

Sarah, a clinical child psychologist, heard about this finding and decided to try it on her twins, Benjamin and Ethan, who were still not sleeping through the night at four months. Sarah had breast-fed her twins for the first three and a half months, usually wearing a favorite nursing nightgown that had two front slits so that she could nurse both twins at the same time. Sarah cut two large squares out of this soft flannel. She placed one in each baby's crib. The babies instantly bonded to this well-known material that was associated with their mother. At fifteen months, Benjamin and Ethan still don't go anywhere without their "blankies," especially to bed.

Your baby may already have gravitated toward a favorite object. Don recalls when his daughter Stephanie fell in love with her new-found friend. In a toy store one day, she emphatically pointed to a soft and cuddly dog. Don handed it to her. He said it was like watching someone fall in love. She stroked it and hugged it, beaming all the while. Since that day, Stephanie won't go anywhere without "Doggie." Such a profound experience may not happen to your child, but you may find a favorite item that she finds soothing. If not, don't force the issue. Some children never develop a strong association with one particular item. In fact, some children relish choosing a different item to take to bed with them every night.

Managing Your Child's Lovey

At some point, many parents worry whether their child will ever give up dragging his lovey with him wherever he goes (think of the *Peanuts* character Linus, with his beloved blanket). There is no need to fret. These transitions usually go more smoothly than expected. There is also no need to rush it. No child has ever started high school dragging his blanket along behind him, although many college students still have their childhood blanket in their dorm room. Most children will naturally start to transition away from their attachment object, needing it with them less and less. Other children, as they get older, may need a little push to start the process. It is best to make the transition slowly. For example, if carrying a teddy bear around at preschool is not appropriate, have your child start by keeping it in his cubby or in his knapsack. This way it's nearby during the day, providing comfort. A next step, which may not happen for a long time, is to leave the bear in the car so that he can wave good-bye to it at drop-off and have a warm reunion with it at the end of the day. A third step may be to leave it on his bed, so it's waiting when he gets home. There is no reason to push your child to give up his object entirely. A teddy bear to sleep with can be comforting to a child (or adult!) of any age.

Crib Safety

A significant number of children are injured and even killed each year in crib accidents. Every year there are approximately 11,500 crib-related injuries that require hospital treatment. The Consumer Product Safety Commission estimates that approximately fifty children die each year because of unsafe cribs (typically older, previously used cribs). Prior to the institution of current crib standards, there were 240 deaths a year.

To protect your child, the Consumer Product Safety Commission developed these guidelines on crib safety. All cribs should have:

✦ A firm, tight-fitting mattress so a baby cannot get trapped between the mattress and the crib.
✦ No missing, loose, broken, or improperly installed screws, brackets, or other hardware on the crib or mattress support.

- No more than 2⅜ inches (about the width of a soda can) between crib slats so that a baby's body cannot fit through the slats; no missing or cracked slats.
- No corner posts over ¹⁄₁₆ inch high so a baby's clothing cannot get caught and lead to strangulation.
- No cutouts in the headboard or footboard so a baby's head cannot get trapped.

Only use a crib that has been manufactured since 1990 and has been certified to meet national safety standards. These cribs will have a Juvenile Products Manufacturers label. If you have a used crib that does not have this label or is not safe, don't use it.

In addition:

- Keep the crib away from radiators, heating vents, and window-blind strings.
- Always keep the side locked in its top position whenever your baby is in the crib.
- Once your baby can sit up, lower the mattress to its lowest setting.
- Keep all pillows and comforters out of the crib to avoid suffocation.
- If you cover your baby with a blanket, place your baby "feet to foot" in the crib. That is, place your baby's feet at the bottom of the crib with the blanket tucked in around the end of the mattress.

And, always place your baby to sleep on his or her back at night and during naptimes.

YOUR BABY'S BEDROOM AND NIGHTCLOTHES

Many parents have questions about their baby's bedroom. Should it be warm or cool? What type of blanket should be on the bed? Should my baby wear an undershirt with his "feetie" pajamas? Should he sleep on one of those sheepskin mattress pads that look so comfy?

Pillows

"When should I give my baby a pillow? She always likes to use one when she is on my bed or the couch. I just don't know whether to put one in her crib."

There are no hard-and-fast rules as to when to give your child a pillow. Pillows are not recommended for children under two years of age because they can easily smother. If you give your child a pillow while he is still in his crib, give him one that is small, the size of an airline pillow. Make sure that it is not too soft and squishy. A feather pillow is not recommended, again because of concerns about smothering. Many parents give their child his first pillow when they move him from a crib to a bed. It just seems that a bed should have a pillow. You should remember, however, that your child doesn't need to have a pillow at this time. Use your own judgment and give him a pillow when you are both ready.

First of all, there are no absolute right answers to any of these questions. You know your baby and your living environment best. The rule of thumb is to dress your baby as you would dress yourself. If you would sleep wearing only a nightshirt under a lightweight blanket, then don't have your baby sleep with an undershirt, heavy pajamas, blanket, and comforter. Young babies do best in an undershirt and pajamas with feet. A lightweight blanket is appropriate, depending on the temperature. Babies notoriously kick off their covers but, unlike you, are unable to cover themselves again. So make sure that your baby is dressed warmly enough to compensate if he becomes uncovered during the night. The best recommendation:

Rather than use a blanket, which can be dangerous anyway because of a risk of suffocation, have your child sleep in a blanket sleeper (those flannel-weight feetie pajamas) or in a sleep sack.

Your baby's bedroom should be toward the cool side of comfortable. Studies have shown that people sleep best in cooler bedrooms compared to warmer bedrooms. Also, being overheated has been identified as a risk factor for SIDS. This does not mean that you should make your baby's bedroom cold. If prior to having a baby you turned your heat way down in the house at night to conserve energy (and money!) and kept warm under numerous blankets, you will need to curtail this severe temperature change. Lower the heat a few degrees if necessary, but don't let the house get too cold. Again, use your judgment.

In terms of your baby's bedding, avoid those comfy-looking sheepskin mattress covers or down covers that go over the mattress. They may look comfortable, but they can be dangerous to your baby, as he can suffocate in the soft surface. In young babies, these will also increase the risk of SIDS (see Chapter 12). Babies should sleep on a firm surface, which reduces their chance of suffocating.

Reminders

- ✦ A set bedtime is important to establishing good sleep habits.
- ✦ A bedtime routine is the key to sleeping through the night.
- ✦ A transitional object, such as a teddy bear or favorite blanket, can make the transition to sleep easier for your child.
- ✦ Ensure that your child's crib is safety-approved.

CHAPTER 6

Sleeping Through the Night: Bedtime Struggles and Night Wakings

Every night Jenny rocks her daughter, Megan, eleven months, to sleep at 7:45 while giving her a bottle. Usually, Megan is fast asleep within fifteen minutes. Megan wakes up at least once every night, sometimes up to three or four times. When she wakes, she cries, looks disoriented, and sits up. Her parents go into her room, pick her up, and give her a bottle, and she instantly falls back to sleep. The whole process takes less than five minutes.

Bernadette begins the process of putting Robert, nineteen months, to bed at 8:00. She is lucky if he is asleep by 9:00. Bernadette rocks Robert to sleep while sitting in a rocking chair. Once he is asleep, she tries to put him in his crib. If she doesn't wait long enough, Robert wakes up and starts to cry. When this happens, she has to start the process all over again. She has gotten to the point where she will sit with him asleep in her arms for twenty to thirty minutes for fear that if she moves he will wake up. During the night, Robert wakes at least twice. Each time Bernadette has to rock him back to sleep. This can take up to thirty minutes.

Clare has tried everything. Her daughter, Roslyn, will not go to sleep at night. For the first year and a half Clare would bounce Roslyn to sleep while pacing the floor. It was a good night if Roslyn was asleep within one hour. At the age of two, Clare switched Roslyn from a crib to a bed, thinking that would solve the problem, because Roslyn screamed every time she was put in her crib. Now, at two and a half, Clare has to lie down with Roslyn on her bed until Roslyn falls asleep. In order for Clare to finally get out of Roslyn's room without waking her daughter, she has to slither off the bed and slowly crawl across the floor, hoping that Roslyn won't wake and catch her. About two hours later, Roslyn wakes up crying and goes into her parents' bedroom. Clare is so tired at that point that it is easier to simply let Roslyn sleep with her for the rest of the night.

Although these three children seem to have very different sleep problems, actually they all have the same underlying problem. Each child needs his parent or some other type of help to fall asleep. This chapter reviews why babies and toddlers have sleep problems and how to get your baby to sleep easily and quickly and assure that he sleeps through the night.

BEDTIME STRUGGLES

There are many reasons that your child may resist going to bed at night, and there are different solutions for each one. The following is a list of the most common reasons and what to do about them.

STAYING UP LATER. Children love evening activities. They get to spend time with their parents, which is especially nice if either or both work during the day. They get to play with their brothers and sisters. They may get to watch television. In going to bed, they miss the fun. By arguing, dawdling, crying, or pleading, they get to stay up later and do fun things.

Leonard and Tammy, for example, insisted that their two-year-old daughter, Mary, just wasn't tired at night. When they put her in her crib, she would stand there, holding on to the railing, crying for them. After about fifteen minutes, they would go get her, give her

Oreo cookies, and let her watch cartoons with them. Why wouldn't she want to stay up if she got to watch television and eat cookies with her favorite people?

The best way to deal with this common bedtime problem is to be firm in setting limits. Have lots of fun in the evening, but bedtime is bedtime. Do not allow your child to get out of bed once you decide it is time for her to go to sleep. Obviously, you can put a child to bed but you can't make her sleep. If she is not tired, she can play by herself in her crib or bed. She can have her favorite toy or book. Whatever you do, though, don't reinforce (i.e., reward) her for not going to sleep. Don't let her go downstairs to play or give her treats. You will only prolong the problem, denying her much-needed sleep and yourself the time that you need at night.

GETTING ATTENTION. Many children find it fun to get out of bed. Each time they get up, they get some extra time to spend with you, and they get to see what is going on in the house. The more you argue, demand, or plead to get your child to bed, the more you are reinforcing your child's bedtime resistance behavior. Don't get sucked into giving bad attention for bad behavior. It is better to give good attention for good behavior. (For a reminder of the difference between good attention and bad attention, see Chapter 3.) In a neutral and calm manner, return your child to his own bed. Don't spend too much time doing it. Be firm and consistent. Another way to deal with these problems is to tell your child that if he is quiet and stays in bed you will come and check on him in five minutes, or three minutes, or whatever interval is appropriate. Make sure you do check on him. This way you will be providing your child with attention for engaging in good behavior. This strategy keeps many a wayward child in his own bed. Often your child will fall asleep while waiting for you to reappear.

SLEEP ASSOCIATIONS. Poor sleep associations are usually the most common reason for infant and toddler sleep problems. The rest of this chapter will focus on what these sleep associations are and how to deal with them.

SLEEP ASSOCIATIONS

Sleep associations are those things or behaviors that are present when we fall asleep. Everyone has associations with falling asleep. As adults, these associations are deeply ingrained. For example, Scott always changes his clothes, brushes his teeth, and reads in bed for at least ten minutes before turning out the light. He always turns a fan on for the constant background noise and closes the bedroom door halfway. He sleeps on his back with two pillows and one light-weight blanket. His wife, Ellen, goes to bed later than Scott. She undresses and takes a shower before going to bed. The sound of the rushing water relaxes her and makes her sleepy. She then turns out all the lights in the house and stumbles her way to bed, being sure not to wake Scott. She removes the second pillow from her side of the bed, gets under the lightweight blanket that also covers Scott and the two extra blankets on her side of the bed, and rolls over onto her stomach.

Scott and Ellen have very different sleep associations. Scott has to read before being able to fall asleep, and Ellen showers. Each sleeps in a different position with a different number of pillows and blankets. Think about your own sleep patterns. What do you do every night before going to bed? Is it relatively the same every night?

As I've said in previous chapters, babies and adults alike wake up during the night. Whatever sleep associations are present for you at bedtime also need to be there for you during the night. If the sleep association is present when you waken, you return to sleep instantly. You may notice one of these arousals if you watch some-one sleep. He may roll over, change position, or simply scratch his face. He doesn't even appear to wake up. If the sleep association is not present, however, he will wake up and try to rectify the situa-tion. If your blanket fell off the bed, you would pick it up. If the hall light was turned on after you went to sleep, you would get up, turn the light off, and go back to sleep. If you do need to get out of bed, you may be awake for a while afterward, unable to return to sleep quickly. Many people think that they wake up because their blanket fell on the floor or the light woke them up. The opposite is true. They woke up naturally, but the blanket being gone or the light being on makes it impossible to fall back to sleep.

Babies, too, have sleep associations, either positive ones or negative ones. Positive sleep associations help babies fall asleep on their own, whether at naptime, bedtime, or during the night. Negative sleep associations are those that babies can't control on their own. They require the presence of something or someone to help them fall asleep. Think about what your baby always does or needs to fall asleep. How do you get your baby to fall asleep?

Positive Sleep Associations

Positive sleep associations are what you want your baby to have in order to help him fall asleep quickly and easily on his own. They should also be present when he wakes during the night. Appropriate positive sleep associations include sleeping in a certain position, sleeping with a teddy bear or favorite object, having the lights off and the door closed, or having a fan running all night. Whatever the association may be in your baby's particular case, the important thing is having the bedroom environment constant at bedtime and throughout the night.

Negative Sleep Associations

Negative sleep associations require your presence or are things that will not be present when your baby wakes up in the middle of the night. Nursing or drinking from a bottle to fall asleep is probably one of the most common negative sleep associations. You will know this is one of your baby's negative associations if you need to feed her to get her to go to sleep. Do you need to feed her again when she wakes in the night in order to get her to return to sleep? Being rocked to sleep is another common sleep association that interferes with a baby's ability to self-soothe back to sleep. Being sung to, cuddled, or having music playing may be what your baby requires to fall asleep. Whatever the association, a negative one interferes with your baby's being able to fall asleep on her own.

WHAT CAUSES NIGHT WAKINGS?

All babies and adults wake throughout the night, anywhere from two to six times. There doesn't have to be any particular reason other than going from one sleep stage to another. Waking is not the problem. The problem occurs when your baby can't soothe herself and fall back to sleep. Instead she needs to be rocked or nursed back to sleep, or she needs music playing or her blankets adjusted. Your goal, therefore, is to create a situation in which your baby can fall back to sleep on her own.

In the beginning, your baby probably went back to sleep quickly once you rocked her or handed her a pacifier. Hopefully, that is still the case. But some children begin to stay awake for longer and longer periods. The reason for these prolonged wakings is that your child realizes what is happening. The moment she falls asleep, you stop nursing her, put her in her crib, and leave. If you were told that the minute you fell asleep someone was going to take your pillow or blanket away, you would resist falling asleep, not wanting to lose your pillow or blanket. Your child is doing the same thing. She will fight falling asleep so that she will not lose her sleep association.

Your baby may also seem angry in the middle of the night when she awakens. She is upset because she is tired and wants to go back to sleep. You would be angry too if every night you woke up in the middle of the night and couldn't go back to sleep until someone got you a drink of water or straightened your blankets for you.

To put it bluntly:

+ If you rock your child to sleep, then every time she wakes up, including the middle of the night, she'll need to be rocked in order to go back to sleep.
+ If you nurse your child to sleep, every time she wakes up, she'll need to nurse in order to go back to sleep.
+ If you sing your child to sleep, whenever she wakes up, she'll need you to sing in order to go back to sleep.

Thus, most babies' problems with sleep are the result of negative sleep associations.

RESEARCH EVIDENCE

Data from multiple sources all support the understanding that sleep associations are the primary reason for bedtime difficulties and nighttime awakenings in young children. Many studies have been published that consistently find that babies who are put to bed awake and soothe themselves to sleep, sleep better than babies who are put to bed already asleep. Yet the recent National Sleep Foundation *Sleep in America* poll found that more than half of all infants (54 percent) are put to bed already asleep. These infants take longer to fall asleep, are twice as likely to wake at night, and sleep on average one hour less at night! It really does make a difference. A baby who soothes himself to sleep will sleep better.

Many studies have been conducted supporting the efficacy of the sleep-training method outlined below. This method, formerly referred to as "graduated extinction" in the medical and psychological literature, has been delineated as well established according to evidence-based guidelines. Multiple sources have come to this conclusion.

THE BASIC BEDTIME METHOD

The basic bedtime method below is based on the concept of replacing your baby's negative sleep associations with positive sleep associations. Unfortunately, this can be a trying process for a few days until new associations are established. A step-by-step guide is provided here to help you through this process.

+ **Step one: Set bedtime**. Step one is to have a set time for your baby to go to bed (see more about bedtimes in Chapter 5). Your baby needs to go to bed at the same time every night. This is important to help set your baby's internal clock so that his body is accustomed to falling asleep at exactly the same time every day. In addition, babies relish routine, and routine is based on the same things happening at the same times every day. Bedtime is bedtime.

+ **Step two: Bedtime routine**. Step two is to establish a consistent bedtime routine. As discussed in Chapter 5, a set bedtime routine is essential to your child's being able to fall asleep easily and quickly. It helps your child get sleepy and get ready for the transition from daytime to sleep time. The end of your child's bedtime routine should be done in your child's room so that he perceives it as a place where positive things happen, rather than as a place where he is sent to go to sleep. Read the last book, have the last cuddle, or sing the last song in his bedroom. The reading, cuddling, and singing should end, though, *before* your child falls asleep.

+ **Step three: Bedroom environment**. This step requires you to spend some time in your child's room during the evening to figure out what it is going to be like for your child when he wakes during the night. What you want to

do is establish a consistent bedroom environment that is
the same at bedtime and throughout the night. Stand in
your child's room. Imagine that it is 2:00 in the morning.
What does your child see? Is a light on in the hallway? Is
music playing? Are you there? Are there toys in bed with
him? If you intend to have music playing all night, then
play music at bedtime. If there is to be no music playing
during the night, then there should be none at bedtime,
because you don't want music to be your child's negative
sleep association. One thing that may help you with this
step is to consider what your child's negative sleep associations may be. What is it that you need to do at bedtime
or in the middle of the night to get your child to sleep?
Do you need to refill a cup of water that is placed beside
his bed? Do you need to turn a night-light on? Do you
have to sing to him? Whatever it may be, either eliminate it altogether or make sure that it is always there.
Again, you need to make sure that your child's bedroom
is the same all the time when he is sleeping.

✦ **Step four: Put down awake**. Now it is time to teach your
child to fall asleep on his own. Yes, this is the hard part.
After your child's bedtime routine is done, put him in his
crib or bed, say good night, and leave the room. Don't
nurse him. Don't let him fall asleep in the living room.
Don't stay with him. Have your child fall asleep alone in
his crib or bed. Your child is likely to be upset by the
change in his routine. He will probably call for you, cry,
or scream. Most likely he will do all three at once. Wait.
Then do a simple checking routine. Go back into your
child's room. Tell him that it is okay. Tell him again that
it is time for him to go to sleep. Pat him or touch him
briefly if you wish. Don't pick him up. Don't cuddle him.
Be gentle but firm. Remain fairly neutral and stay for a
brief time, no more than one minute. Basically, make the

visits brief and boring. You don't want to reinforce your child's crying by staying long or giving him too much attention. That is, you don't want to make it worth his while to cry for you. Leave. Wait again. Check again. Repeatedly wait and then check on your child. This could take a while.

How long should you wait before checking on your child? Check on your child as frequently or infrequently as you wish. It depends entirely on your tolerance level and your child's temperament. Some parents can't bear to listen to their child cry for more than thirty seconds. That is okay. Start there. Wait only thirty seconds. Then continue to check as frequently as you wish. The longer you can wait, the better, but it doesn't really matter. Some children get more upset seeing their parents than if left alone. If this is the case, wait longer periods rather than shorter ones. Remember, the goal is not to make your child upset, but to have your child fall asleep on his own. All you want is that golden moment when your child falls asleep independently. How you get there doesn't really matter.

How long should it take until your child finally falls asleep? Most children cry for about forty-five minutes the first night. On the second night, expect it to last longer, about an hour, as if your child is saying, "Look, last night must have been a fluke. Tonight I really mean it." In clinical terms this is known as an "extinction burst" (for more about this, see Chapter 3). On the third night expect about twenty minutes. Bottom line: you can expect your child to be going to bed easily and quickly within the week. Keep in mind, though, that there are some children—those who are strong-willed—who will cry longer, even for an hour or two on those first few nights.

If your child has been crying for a very long time, you can take a break. Go get her, take a walk around the house, read another story, and then try again. You don't want to rescue her completely by returning to your old habits of nursing or rocking her to sleep. Doing so will simply teach your child to cry for long periods. But if you absolutely need to, take a few minutes to calm everyone down, and then put her back down again. And, obviously, if you think that there is a problem, go in and check on your child. Don't feel that you absolutely must wait.

Your child's resistance is normal and understandable. Think about it: It would take you a few days to adjust if you were required to establish new sleep associations, such as learning to sleep without a pillow or without a blanket. Some people also find it difficult to make the transition to sleeping someplace new, such as in a hotel room or at a friend's house. Here you are changing all the rules on your child, so expect it to take a few days to a week until the new sleep associations take hold. In fact, once your child is falling asleep quickly at bedtime, don't be surprised if sleep problems return for a short period. This doesn't mean that the sleep training was ineffective. Remain consistent in your efforts, and your baby will again be falling asleep quickly and sleeping through the night.

WHAT TO DO IF YOUR CHILD
WAKES DURING THE NIGHT

Do what you normally do! If you usually rock your baby back to sleep during the night, then go ahead and rock her. If you usually nurse or take her to your bed, then do that. Research has found that once a baby is falling asleep quickly and easily at bedtime, then she'll naturally start sleeping through the night in about two weeks. This is the case for about 80 percent of all children. Why? Because once your baby has the skill of being able to fall asleep on her own, she'll start doing it at all times. It's just like learning to crawl. If your baby learns to crawl in the morning, she'll be able to do it in the afternoon. If she learns to fall asleep on her own at bedtime, she'll be able to do it in the middle of the night.

In the meantime, do what you normally do when your baby wakes up in the middle of the night. If you usually rock her back to sleep, then rock her. If you pace the floor, then pace. Gradually, as your baby learns to self-soothe when she initially falls asleep at bedtime, she will begin to put herself back to sleep more often during the middle of the night.

This process does not happen immediately, however, and there will be night wakings during the first few weeks. Responding to your baby at these times is better than letting her cry in the middle of the night and will not interfere with her learning to put herself to sleep. Also, it will ensure that you respond to your child's needs during the night. So for everyone's sanity and so everyone can get as much sleep as possible, do whatever it takes to get your child back to sleep during the night.

The key is to continue to follow the basic bedtime method at bedtime! If your child still continues to wake after several weeks of falling asleep easily and quickly at bedtime, see Chapter 10 for what to do.

THE STORY OF MAX

Sally and Richard arrived at the office, looking exhausted, carrying their fourteen-month-old son, Max. Since the day they brought him home, Max had never slept through the night. Each night either Sally or Richard would rock Max to sleep at bedtime. A few hours later, usually around midnight and again around 3:30 a.m., Max would wake up, and either Sally or Richard would rock him back to sleep. On a good night this took only about five to ten minutes. On some nights, an hour or two would pass before Max would go back to sleep. Neither Sally nor Richard thought things would ever change.

After much discussion about sleep and positive and negative sleep associations, Sally and Richard realized that they needed to teach Max how to fall asleep on his own. A bedtime routine that was comfortable for them was mapped out. Max's bedtime was set for 7:30, and his parents began a soothing bedtime routine around 7:00. Pajamas were put on, stories that Max loved to hear were read, and at 7:30 Max was put in his crib with his favorite teddy bear and his parents kissed him good night. Max's parents would check on him every five minutes to make sure that he was fine and to reassure Max that they were nearby.

Sally and Richard were warned that on the first night it would take Max about forty minutes to fall asleep, on the second night about an hour (a usual occurrence), and by the third night Max would probably be asleep within twenty minutes. Once Max began to fall asleep on his own at bedtime, he would know how to fall back to sleep naturally when he awakened in the middle of the night.

Sally and Richard went home determined to solve Max's sleep problems and get him to sleep through the night. That night, Sally received an emergency call from work, so they scrapped their sleep plans. Since it was a Wednesday night, they decided to wait for the weekend so they would feel less pressured by work concerns when they started Max on his new program. On Friday night Sally and Richard agreed that Richard would take on bedtime duty that first night because he felt more prepared to deal with Max's being upset. At 7:00, Richard announced that it was bedtime. He and Max had fun getting ready for bed. Richard sang while getting Max ready for bed, played his favorite peekaboo game with him, and read Max some of his favorite stories. All was fine until Richard put Max in his crib. After looking stunned for a few moments, Max began to cry. Richard told him that everything was okay and left the room, feeling that his heart was breaking as Max continued to cry. Richard waited five minutes and went to check on Max. Again, he told him that everything was okay and it was time to go to sleep. Five minutes later Richard checked again. Seven minutes later Richard couldn't wait any longer and checked again. Seeing that Max was getting more upset when he went in, Richard waited ten minutes the next time. Finally, after exactly fifty-two minutes, Max fell asleep holding his teddy bear and looking exhausted. Max wakened twice that night, and each time Richard rocked him back to sleep.

On Saturday night Sally put Max to bed. She did the same bedtime routine that Richard had done the night before. When it was time to put Max in his crib, he got upset immediately. Sally reassured him and gingerly left the room. At the five-minute mark, Max was sobbing and reaching up to Sally when she went in to check on him. He finally fell asleep after an hour and a quarter.

On the third night Sally and Richard flipped a coin to determine who was going to handle bedtime. Neither was looking forward to another night of crying. To their surprise, Max didn't begin crying until after they had been gone for about five minutes. They waited another five minutes before checking on him. Within fifteen minutes Max was sound asleep. The next few nights went similarly, with Max crying less and less. For that first week Max continued to wake during the night and needed to be rocked back to sleep. A few times, though, they heard him whimper and go back to sleep on his own.

Although the first few nights were difficult, Sally and Richard reassured themselves that they were doing the right thing. Two weeks later, Richard commented that "it feels like a miracle." He couldn't believe it. Life was completely different. Max was going to bed at 7:30, falling asleep quickly, and not waking up again until 7:00 the next morning. Sally and Richard were enjoying life again, and Max was happier than he usually was during the day. Sally and Richard knew that they were likely to encounter problems again with Max's sleep if they went on vacation or if he became sick, but they felt that they knew how to take control and help Max to fall asleep on his own and return to sleeping through the night.

DRINKING FROM A BOTTLE OR NURSING

As mentioned previously, many babies fall asleep while drinking from a bottle or nursing. These children all have a negative sleep association that is preventing them from falling asleep on their own. Another reason why many children who breast-feed or bottle-feed at bedtime and in the middle of the night do not sleep through the night is that they awaken with a soaked diaper. All of those fluids have to go somewhere! Almost all children over the age of six months no longer need nighttime feedings. If you think that your baby needs a final bottle or nursing time, move it to earlier in the evening and break the association of feeding with sleep. Nurse your baby thirty to sixty minutes earlier and then have playtime before bedtime. Or at least move it to earlier in the bedtime routine.

If your baby associates nursing or drinking from a bottle with sleeping, you will need to change this negative sleep association to a positive one. The method that will accomplish this is similar to the basic bedtime method, but rather than stop the feeding abruptly, it will be easier on you and your baby if you do it gradually.

The Bottle Feeder

The easiest way to get your baby from requiring a bottle to fall asleep at bedtime is to wean him off it by reducing the amount of liquid in the bedtime bottle by one ounce every night or every other night. Use the sample tables below as a guide, depending on the amount you normally give your baby.

As you can see, if your baby usually drinks an eight-ounce bottle at bedtime, then your baby will be off his bottle by the seventh night. If you are starting with a four-ounce bottle, then the process will take only five nights. If your baby protests for more

Weaning from a Bottle at Bedtime

Night	Starting with an 8-oz. bottle
Night 1	7 oz.
Night 2	6 oz.
Night 3	5 oz.
Night 4	4 oz.
Night 5	3 oz.
Night 6	2 oz.
Night 7	No bottle

Night	Starting with a 4-oz. bottle
Night 1	3 oz.
Night 2	3 oz.
Night 3	2 oz.
Night 4	2 oz.
Night 5	No bottle

milk, hang in there and just rock or hold him until he is asleep. You will notice that giving a one-ounce bottle is not recommended. This is because a one-ounce bottle can be a tease to your child and may just make him more upset than having no bottle at all. When you get to no bottle at bedtime, continue to hold him or rock him to sleep. Definitely expect a few rough nights, but then you will be over the hump.

Once you are rid of the bottle and your baby is able to fall asleep easily without it at bedtime, then it is time to move on to the above basic bedtime method. Start putting your child down to sleep when he is awake. Again, having your child put himself to sleep is the key to getting a good night's sleep.

The Breast Feeder

You can use a similar technique for weaning your child off of bed-time nursing, although it is harder. Since you cannot tell how much milk your child gets when nursing, use the number of minutes that he is nursing as your measure. For the first few nights, simply time how long your baby nurses at bedtime. Once you have that informa-tion, you can start to wean him gradually. Decrease the number of minutes your child nurses by one minute per night. Other mothers have done this by popping their baby off the breast earlier and ear-lier, before the baby is fast asleep. So, each night, have him stop nursing when he is more and more wide-awake.

Rather than slowly cutting back the nursing-to-sleep time, it may be easier simply to move nursing to earlier in the bedtime rou-tine and then rock your baby to sleep. Move nursing to a different room and then do your baby's bedtime routine in his room or nurse in your baby's room and then add a final step, such as changing into pajamas or reading a story. If you, the mother, are going to be the one to rock your baby to sleep after nursing, it may be better to stand and walk your baby to sleep, as you won't be in nursing posi-tion. Another, easier, way is to have someone else take over after nursing to rock the baby to sleep.

Similarly, if you are trying to cut out nursing during the night or when you start sleep training it is often best if the nursing mother is not the one who does the training process. It is almost like teasing a baby with the proximity of the breast and milk: "Here they are, but you can't have them." Try to get someone else to put the baby down and to check on him every few minutes. You, Mom, can still do your baby's bedtime routine, of course, but leave the last good night to someone else. After your baby has started to get the hang of falling asleep on his own, you can start putting him to bed again. Expect a minor flare-up at this point, since your baby will probably think that his favorite activity of nursing will resume. Continue to do your usual checking routine if he is upset. But in a few days your baby will start going to sleep quickly and easily for you as well.

DEALING WITH AN OLDER CHILD

If your child is a little older, i.e., toddler age and above, other methods to help her sleep through the night can be employed. Most of these require that your child understand language, have some sense of time, and have a bit of patience.

Stay Shorter and Shorter

Rather than leave your child alone for longer and longer periods of time, you can stay with your child for shorter and shorter periods. Cynthia and Ray did this with their three-year-old daughter, Karley. At night either Cynthia or Ray had to stay with Karley until she was just about asleep. After reading stories to her and getting her a last drink of water, they usually ended up staying with Karley for about twenty minutes. For the first two nights Cynthia stayed with Karley for the entire twenty minutes, but rather than wait quietly and leave when Karley was just about asleep, she told Karley after fifteen minutes that she would be staying for five more minutes. At the five-minute mark, she kissed her good night one last time and left. On the third and fourth nights she stayed a total of fifteen minutes, telling Karley after ten minutes that she was staying another five minutes. On night five Cynthia stayed a total of ten minutes, and on night six she stayed only five minutes. Each time she told Karley she would be staying five more minutes.

When using this technique, it is helpful to emphasize the positive. Cynthia always made sure that she told Karley she would be staying five more minutes; she didn't tell her she would be leaving in five minutes. Setting a timer for five minutes can also be beneficial. This way the timer says that you have to leave, rather than it appearing ar-bitrary. You won't get into arguments about "just one more minute."

Run Errands

One difficulty many children have at bedtime is that they do not want to be left alone. Your child may need practice before she is ready to be left alone cold turkey. As your child gets older, she will begin to understand time and the concept that if you leave, you will return. Use this knowledge to your advantage. Run errands. First, go get a drink or get something from another room. Tell her, "Oops, Daddy forgot his glasses. I'll be right back." In the beginning, if your child has never been left alone in her room at nighttime, leave for very short periods of time, less than twenty seconds. Then start running errands that take longer. Go to another part of the house to get something. Go fold laundry or load the dishwasher. Clean the bath-room. Your child will get practice at being alone—and you will get some chores done. Make each errand last longer and longer. You can begin with one errand a night or do a few each night. Each time you return, praise your child for staying in her room alone. Tell her how good she is and how much you appreciate her staying in her bed or crib. The key to this strategy is that you must return even if she falls asleep. Don't forget. Set a timer. Don't be distracted by the phone or the television. If you forget just one time, it will encour-age your child to call for you or, worse, to come get you to make sure that you have not forgotten her.

"I'll Be Back"

What your child wants is your attention, and most of the time he will cry to get it. But you can turn this situation around. Set up a scenario in which your child needs to be quiet and in bed in order to get your attention. After you say good night, tell him that you will be back in five minutes and give him another kiss good night if he is quiet and in bed. Leave the room and then come back in five minutes. Again, the key is that you have to return! It is harder to remember to return than when doing errands, because there is no distinct end point to what you are doing. So to make this work, set a timer. When the timer goes off, go check on your child. Give him another kiss good night and tell him how good he is being. Some children require a shorter interval than five minutes, so return after two or three minutes. You can even set the timer for just thirty seconds if that is all you think your child can handle. Should you do this again a second or third time in one night? Yes, if you think it will help. For some children just one "I'll be back" is sufficient, but other children will need to see you again. Some children will fall asleep before you get back, but you still must return. You want to tell the truth the next morning if he asks if you came back. He may also be only half asleep waiting for you, so don't postpone or cancel your check-in.

Sleep Fairy

Older toddlers also do very well responding to rewards. Sticker charts can be very effective, although children typically need to be three years or older to understand sticker charts. Preschoolers, especially, will do almost anything for a sticker. Set it up so that your child will be successful in getting a sticker. Start with small, attainable goals, such as sleeping in her own bed all night, rather than larger, more difficult goals, such as sleeping through the night without ever calling out for you. Stickers can be redeemed for small prizes every day or two. Prizes should be small and family-oriented, such as a trip to the library or a family bike ride.

Sleep fairies can also be highly motivating. The sleep fairy comes in and leaves a present under a child's pillow if she's done a good job at bedtime or during the night. The present can be something like a sticker. Andrea had the sleep fairy leave a penny under her daughter's pillow every night. As she said, "sleep is definitely worth $3.65 a year."

OTHER METHODS

There are other methods that can be used to resolve your child's sleeping problems. Remember, though, that the basic bedtime method and its variations are tried and true. Much research has supported its effectiveness. If you do it and follow through, your child will be going to sleep on his own within a week and sleeping through the night within two to three weeks.

Below, however, are some other strategies that you may wish to try.

THE SLOWER APPROACH: GRADUAL PARENT REMOVAL. Some parents are unable to tolerate their child's being upset at bedtime (but see Chapter 9 on how to cope). An alternative approach is to ease yourself gradually out of your child's presence. Start with sitting in a chair or on the floor by your child's crib or bed. Stay there until he falls asleep. After two to three nights of this, move your chair a little farther away: two to three feet away for nights three and four, and then several more feet away for nights five and six. On the seventh night you should be sitting in the doorway. On night nine, move into the hallway. Within ten days to two weeks your child should be falling asleep on his own.

JUST LET HIM CRY. Some people recommend just letting the baby cry as the best way to deal with a baby who won't go to sleep by himself. Other parents you know may say this; your own parents may say this; even your pediatrician may suggest it. You can try it. It can work. It can also backfire. For instance, you may be ignoring your child when he really needs you. It would be horrible not to go in and check on him and later find that his foot is caught in the crib rails or that something else has happened to him. Another drawback is that you may not be able to tolerate it. After about fifteen minutes to an hour of hearing him crying, you may give in and pick him up. Then you will have made the problem worse: you will have taught him that if he cries long enough and hard enough, you will come to get him. Next time, he will cry even louder and for a longer time, expecting that eventually you will give in.

Another potential problem is that children who are allowed to cry it out seem to cry for a longer time before finally falling asleep and sometimes are unable to settle themselves down. Rather than falling asleep after forty minutes, they may cry for over an hour or even two hours. This makes it harder on everyone. So give this method a try if you want to; just be forewarned of the pitfalls.

MEDICATIONS. Some pediatricians recommend or prescribe Benadryl or chloral hydrate to help babies sleep. Does it work? Is this a good idea?

Research has shown that some medications do decrease the number of times a baby wakes during the night, but this is from a statistical point of view, not from a parent's point of view. Thus, rather than your baby waking an average of 3.2 times per night, she will wake only 2.5 times per night. Statistically, this is a significant reduction, and the conclusion drawn from the study is that the medication worked. For parents, though, this means that rather than waking three times per night, the baby is waking two times on some nights. This is not the solution that most parents want. Your goal is to get your baby to sleep through the night. Therefore, medications are not the answer.

Also, with any medication there is the concern of side effects. These types of sedative medications are not usually harmful to a baby, but they can make her groggy the next day. Another problem with medications is that they change sleep, so your baby may not be getting all the different stages of sleep that she needs.

Finally, medications don't work because they do not resolve the problems of poor sleep associations. Your baby will still need to fall asleep with you rocking her, feeding her, or singing to her. And although she will wake less frequently during the night, she will continue to need you to help her get back to sleep. Once you stop the medication, your baby will go right back to waking as much as she ever did. Some people propose that by giving a baby a sleeping pill for a few days to a few weeks, it will "break the cycle" of the sleep problem. This does not happen. Your baby will simply revert to her old sleeping habits once you stop giving her the medicine.

WHAT DOESN'T WORK: DON'T EVEN BOTHER

There are many things that parents do to attempt to get their baby to sleep. Unfortunately, many of these attempts are futile. Here is a list of what not to bother with, especially since some methods can even backfire and cause more problems.

SOLID FOODS. Some believe that babies wake because they are hungry; therefore, they should be given solid foods at a very young age. No research has supported this belief. Solid foods do not help babies sleep. Remember, all babies wake. It is just a matter of whether or not your baby can put herself back to sleep. Babies who want to eat during the night have become conditioned to do so. By a relatively young age, babies receive all the nutrients they need during the day.

LATER BEDTIME. Parents try to move their baby's bedtime later, hoping he will be so tired that he will fall asleep faster. This doesn't work. When babies get overtired, they get crankier and have a harder time, not an easier time, settling down and falling asleep. Your problems will just get worse if you wait to put your baby down.

ELIMINATING DAYTIME NAPS. In an attempt to get babies to sleep at night, parents try removing daytime naps. Don't bother. Babies need their naps, and if they are denied them, they will be more tired and have more problems falling asleep at night and sleeping throughout the night. Besides, have you ever tried to keep a baby awake when she is determined to fall asleep? It's an almost impossible task. What may also happen is that your sleep-deprived baby will fall asleep at 5:00. Now you are really in trouble, because there is no way she will go to sleep for the night at 7:30.

GROWING OUT OF IT. Babies don't grow out of sleep problems. Studies show that most babies with sleep problems at one year of age will still have sleep problems at four years of age if nothing is done. Regrettably, though, this advice is often given by grandparents, neighbors, friends, and even pediatricians. Don't waste weeks and months of sleepless nights waiting for something that probably won't happen. Do something about it now and relish those nights of sleep ahead.

JUST SHORT-TERM SOLUTIONS, UNFORTUNATELY

Parents try many methods, most of which turn out to be short-term solutions. Remember that what will get your baby to go to sleep quickly may lead to a poor sleep association, and your baby will not be able to fall asleep on her own without the association being present. Consider these examples.

DRIVING IN THE CAR. Parents often find that their baby is likely to fall asleep if they put her in the car and go for a drive. The rhythmic motion of a moving car and the constant noise of the engine lull the baby to sleep. Some parents resort to this on a daily (and nightly) basis. In the short term, it works. In the long term, however, it does not teach your baby how to fall asleep on her own, and you will be doing a lot of driving in the months ahead.

VIBRATING CRIB MECHANISMS. There are several mechanisms on the market advertised as being designed to soothe your baby to sleep. Some simply vibrate the crib. Others vibrate the crib and come with a tape of a mother's heartbeat. These may or may not work for your baby. At this time there is no scientific evidence that these really work. Even if they do, they will help only in the short run, getting your baby to sleep today and tomorrow, but not next week or next month. Remember, your baby needs to learn how to be a self-soother so that he can put himself to sleep at bedtime and throughout the night when he wakes up. A vibrating crib simply instills a negative sleep association.

CONSTANT NOISES. Parents are ingenious at figuring out ways to put a baby to sleep. Placing your baby in a car seat on the dryer while it is running works. If you ever try this, however, do not leave your baby alone! There is a very high likelihood that the car seat will fall off the dryer because of the vibration. Teddy bears that make a noise that mimics the mother's heartbeat fall into the same category. One family referred to their vacuum cleaner as "Betty the Babysitter." They had just moved into a new home and were trying to get it painted. While they were painting, they put their five-week-old baby in a car seat on the floor and turned on the vacuum cleaner. Within moments their baby was asleep, and off they would go to paint.

Again, these things work, but they should be considered only short-term solutions. You do not want to teach your baby that she needs the constant vibration or noise to fall asleep, or you will have to turn the vacuum cleaner on every night at bedtime and do so throughout the night.

SOME IMPORTANT TIPS

TIP ONE: STICK WITH IT. Once you decide to begin to teach your child to fall asleep on his own, don't abandon ship halfway through the process. Once you make a commitment, stick with it. Otherwise, you will only teach your child to scream for a longer time the next time because he will expect you to not follow through.

TIP TWO: ANTICIPATE PITFALLS. Anticipate every pitfall you can so that you have a plan for what to do in different situations. Chapter 10 provides a long list of what to do in many different scenarios, such as if your child tries to jump out of the crib, vomits, or gets undressed. It is important for calm and consistent follow-through that you have a plan for handling different contingencies before you start sleep training.

TIP THREE: HOW TO COPE. The process of teaching your child to be a self-soother and to fall asleep on his own can be stressful. There are many ways to help you, the parent, deal with this stressful event, including blocking out noise, getting help, and using relaxation strategies. Chapter 9 provides numerous suggestions on how to cope.

TIP FOUR: DON'T GET UPSET. When you are in the midst of trying to teach your child to fall asleep on her own, don't get upset with her. Your getting upset will only make things worse. If you are calm, it will help her to be calm. Don't spank your child or yell at her. You need to help her make this transition from negative sleep associations to positive ones. She is not deliberately acting out to get on your nerves. She is tired, and all she wants to do is fall asleep. Keep this in mind when you go in for the seventeenth time or return her to her room for the eighth time. Stay calm and soothing, but neutral.

TIP FIVE: BE CREATIVE. As you begin to develop your own strategy for teaching your baby to fall asleep on his own and to sleep through the night, be creative. Remember, the goal is to achieve that golden moment when your baby falls asleep on his own. Whatever you can do to achieve that, go for it. Some strategies were given above, but you can try different solutions of your own, such as one mom who literally kept picking up her child every minute or two but stuck with it until her child fell asleep in her crib. She picked her up over twenty times the first night, but was much more comfortable doing this than leaving. Figure out what will work best for you and your child. Trust your instincts.

TIP SIX: GIVE LOTS OF ATTENTION. Give your child lots of attention at other times of the day. Often your child is crying or acting up to get your attention. By setting limits on your child's bedtime behavior, it is likely that your child will be receiving less attention overall. This will just make your child want your attention even more. To counteract this, make sure that your child gets more attention at other times. Spend extra time with her in the morning or afternoon. Let her help you make dinner. Make the bedtime routine a longer one: read an extra book or sing an extra song.

TIP SEVEN: WHEN NOT TO TRY. As important as it is for you to help your baby sleep through the night, there are good times and bad times to start this process. The good times are when you will be home for a period of time and things are calm in your life. The bad times are when typical household routines are altered, such as when you are working overtime or your usual child care provider is on vacation.

If you are about to go on vacation, even if you will not be leaving for two to three weeks, wait until you get back to start sleep training. If a holiday is coming up and your baby's schedule is going to become inconsistent, you should wait. If you are about to have overnight visitors, wait until the house returns to normal. If this is a stressful period at work or at home, then wait. If you are about to move, wait until you are settled in your new residence.

MAKE SLEEP TRAINING A SUCCESS

Sleep training works, but in order to make it work for you, tailor it to what you can handle so that both you and your child can be successful. If you need to wait short times, wait short times. Think about the end goal, which is having your child fall asleep on her own in her own crib or bed. There are many ways and steps to get to that point. The basic bedtime method described in this chapter is an intermediate step. There are larger steps and there are smaller steps. Take a step that is right for you and your child.

If you need to make a change quickly, then do sleep training during the night as well as at bedtime. Phyllis, a surgeon who was about to go back to work after maternity leave, was worried about being up many times throughout the night and not being alert enough to do surgery the next day. She needed to do sleep training in one fell swoop. She took three nights, doing the checking method at bedtime and throughout the night. Within a week, her daughter was going down easily and sleeping through the night.

Take smaller steps if you don't mind things going slower. Sit by the crib at bedtime for the first week. Or pick up your child and give her a hug every time you check on her. Once your child is starting to fall asleep easily, then progress to moving out of her room or checking on her but not picking her up.

Bottom line: start with the biggest step that you feel comfortable making and keep taking more and more steps toward the ultimate goal. It is better to choose a small step that you will be successful at than taking a big step and quitting. Think of each step as laying the foundation for the ultimate goal of self-soothing to sleep. If it takes a hundred tiny steps to get you and your child to the finish line, that is better than three giant leaps that end in failure.

WARNING

The hope and belief that most parents have is that they will have to deal with sleep issues only once and that when their baby is sleeping through the night, their worries are over. Unfortunately, this isn't the case. You will almost certainly have to deal with sleep issues again (see Chapter 11 on obstacles to continued good sleep and solutions to these common problems). A child's sleep will be disturbed by illness, vacations, and the development of separation anxiety (an aspect of normal development when your child will not want to be apart from you). There will even be times when your baby won't sleep for no apparent reason. That is the bad news. The good news is that each time your baby's sleep begins to be problematic, if you have a set bedtime routine and put her to bed awake, she will return to sleeping through the night quicker and with less fuss each time.

Reminders

- ✦ There are many reasons that young children resist going to bed, including wanting to stay up later and getting attention.
- ✦ Poor sleep associations are the primary reasons that children have sleep problems.
- ✦ Waking at night is normal; the problem is falling back to sleep.
- ✦ Replace your child's negative sleep associations with positive sleep associations.
- ✦ The basic bedtime method will get your baby going to bed and falling asleep quickly and easily.
- ✦ The basic bedtime method needs to be employed only at bedtime. If your baby wakes during the night, you can respond as usual.
- ✦ Although your child will take longer to fall asleep at bedtime for the first three to five days of using the basic bedtime method, after that your child will start falling asleep quickly at bedtime.
- ✦ Once your child is falling asleep quickly and easily on his own at bedtime, in about two weeks he'll start sleeping through the night.
- ✦ Be creative when teaching older children how to fall asleep on their own.
- ✦ There are other methods to change your child's sleep problems, including gradually removing yourself.
- ✦ Avoid using medications, changing your baby's naptimes or bedtime, or moving your baby to solid foods to solve your child's sleep problems. They won't work.

CHAPTER 7

Peace and Quiet: Naptime

Martina is totally frustrated. Juan, seven months, sleeps great at night, but naps are a complete nightmare. She spends much of the day trying to get him to fall asleep. She'll take him for a stroll, put him in a swing, and bounce him for what feels like hours on end. She's lucky if he'll nap for an hour total throughout the day. It feels as if trying to get Juan to nap has taken over her life.

Charlotte, three years old, naps on some days but not on others. On days that she takes a nap, she won't fall asleep at night until 9:30, compared to her usual 8:00 bedtime. Her parents don't know whether to stop her naps completely to ensure an earlier bedtime or insist on a daily nap and put up with her later bedtime.

NAPTIME BASICS

Parents often have as many questions about naptime as they do about nighttime sleep. There are no hard-and-fast rules about naps, but below are some guidelines.

WHERE SHOULD MY BABY NAP? During the first few months, your newborn will likely sleep anywhere, whether at home or out at the grocery store. This won't last long, though. Once your baby gets older, being out will likely be too stimulating and your baby will be much too interested in the world around him to fall asleep. It's best to have your child nap at home and, more important, in the same place he sleeps during the night. Avoid falling into the habit of having your baby take a nap only in the swing or in the stroller. It may seem fine for the moment, but it won't be fine when your little one is two or three years old and won't nap elsewhere. The earlier you make the transition to naps in the crib (or wherever your little one sleeps at night), the more easily and smoothly it will go.

How long should my baby nap? All children are different, as you will find out in many, many ways. Some babies and toddlers need lots of daytime sleep, while others do not. Parents of fraternal twins often note the difference in how much sleep their babies need. Barbara found that her eight-month-old twins were dramatically different in how well they napped every day and how much sleep each needed. Donovan usually took two naps each day, each lasting at least an hour and a half, whereas she was lucky if she could get Michael to sleep for more than forty-five minutes in the morning and in the afternoon. There are things parents can do to encourage naps (see below), but you can't make a baby fall asleep and stay asleep for a long time.

What time should my baby take a nap? In the first couple of months, your baby will likely take a nap many times throughout the day, often with no set schedule. As your newborn gets a bit older, you can start setting naptimes. Starting around two to three months until about six to nine months, you can follow one of two schedules: you can either set naptimes by the *clock* or by the *two-hour rule*.

If you set naps according to the *clock*, stick to the same time every day. For example, your baby may nap every day at 9:30 a.m. and 2:30 p.m. What time you set will likely be determined by the time your baby usually wakes up in the morning. If you have an early riser, the first nap will be closer to 8:00 or 8:30, and around 9:00 or 9:30 if you have a later riser. The afternoon nap will also shift accordingly. Once your toddler moves to one nap a day, naptime will likely start between 12:30 and 1:30. Once this schedule is established, you will be amazed at how precisely your baby's internal clock will be set to her naptimes. Allison found this to be the case with her two-year-old daughter Annie. Annie took a nap every day at 1:00. On family car trips, whether the family left at 10:00 in the morning or at 1:00 in the afternoon, Annie fell asleep at exactly 1:00. It was uncanny.

If you set naps according to the *two-hour rule*, your baby will take a nap exactly two hours (usually almost to the minute) from when she last woke up. Follow this schedule throughout the day. So if your baby wakes up for the day at 6:35 a.m., her first nap will be at 8:35. If she sleeps for an hour, her next naptime will be at 11:35; however, if she sleeps for two hours, her next nap will be at 12:35. This schedule means less predictability from day to day, but it's amazing how babies on two-hour schedules get sleepy precisely two hours after they last woke up. Note, though, that some young babies are ready for their morning nap one and a half hours after waking up, and every two hours thereafter.

WHAT SHOULD MY BABY'S NAP SCHEDULE BE LIKE? Every baby is different. Some babies take two naps a day, each lasting an hour or two. Other babies will take three naps, each lasting thirty to forty-five minutes. The best way to tell if your baby is getting enough daytime sleep is by whether he seems happy and alert. If he's frequently cranky, try making changes in his nap schedule; otherwise, don't worry about it. Also, there is no rule that says how long your baby must sleep. To gain a sense of the average amount of time young children nap at different ages, see the chart on the next page.

SHOULD I EVER WAKE MY BABY FROM HIS NAP? Absolutely! To keep your baby on schedule, wake him when naptime should be

Average Naptime Durations

	Infants	Toddlers	Preschoolers
No nap	1%	3%	48%
Less than 1 hour	<1%	1%	5%
1 to 2 hours	7%	30%	24%
2 to 3 hours	19%	52%	19%
3 hours or more	73%	14%	4%
Average number of hours	3.8	2.0	1.6

Source: 2004 National Sleep Foundation *Sleep in America* poll

over. For example, Dineen would wake Eric from his morning nap at 11:00 so that he would be ready for his afternoon nap at 2:30. She would also wake him at 4:00 from his afternoon nap so that he would be ready for bedtime at 7:30. Most days she did not need to get him up, but it helped keep him on schedule. It seems crazy to wake a sleeping baby, but it works!

HOW LATE SHOULD MY BABY NAP? Most infants and toddlers shouldn't nap after 4:00 or so, as later napping will make it hard for them to fall asleep at bedtime. Very young babies, however, can often take a late-afternoon nap around 5:00 and still be ready for bed at 7:30.

TRANSITIONING NAPS

There are two major transition times with naps. The first is the change from two naps a day to one nap a day. This change usually occurs between twelve and eighteen months, although it sometimes happens earlier or later. The second major transition occurs when a child stops taking naps altogether. The chart on the next page shows how many naps children take at different ages.

Percentage of Children Taking One, Two, or Three Naps per Day			
	One nap per day	Two naps per day	Three-plus naps per day
0–2 months	4%	16%	76%
3–5 months	9%	34%	55%
6–8 months	10%	61%	29%
9–11 months	11%	75%	11%
12–17 months	60%	40%	
18–23 months	87%	13%	
24–35 months	80%	1%	
3 years	57%		
4 years	26%		
5 years	14%		
6 years	2%		

Source: 2004 National Sleep Foundation *Sleep in America* poll

It's important to understand that these changes do not occur overnight. Rather, there is usually a period from a couple of weeks to even a few months during which a child may need to nap more on some days than others. Don't expect an immediate change.

Transitioning from Two Naps to One Nap

Typically by eighteen months of age, most babies are taking only one afternoon nap. This nap may or may not be the same length as the previous two daily naps. That is, some toddlers who took a one-hour nap both in the morning and the afternoon will move to a two-hour nap in the afternoon. Other toddlers will move to taking only an hour-and-a-half afternoon nap.

WHAT ARE THE SIGNS? Your child will start showing signs that she is ready to move to one nap sometime between one and two years of age. The most common sign is that she will simply stop taking one of the naps. Another sign is that she'll take a much longer time to fall asleep for one (or both) of the naps. A third sign is that on days that she misses her morning nap, she does fine, or she may or may not take a longer afternoon nap.

HOW TO MAKE THE TRANSITION. There are several different ways that you can facilitate the transition. One way is simply to keep your child up in the morning and put her down for an afternoon nap. Another way is to move the morning nap later by about fifteen or thirty minutes every two to three days. Finally, there are some toddlers who are not ready to make the transition in one major leap. For these children, you can alternate between one-nap days and two-nap days. Follow the lead of your child.

WHEN CHILD CARE TRANSITIONS NAPS TOO EARLY. Many child care centers will switch a child to a one-nap schedule when the baby moves to the toddler room. This may occur when the baby turns one, or it can occur at a specified time of the year, such as at the beginning of September, when all children transition together to a new room. However your child care center makes this change, it may be before your child is ready to move to one nap. It is unlikely that your toddler can continue taking two naps at child care, but this doesn't mean that you need to make the switch altogether. When my daughter began child care at fifteen months, she was still taking two naps a day. On those days she was at child care, she took one nap and did fine. The added stimulation of the other children kept her awake and happy in the morning. However, on those days she was home, she continued taking two naps. Thus, she took one nap a day three days a week at school, and two naps a day for the four days a week that she was home or at her grandmother's house. This schedule continued until she was twenty months old, when she was ready to transition to one nap every day. Toddlers are flexible and can tolerate this kind of change in nap schedules.

DEVELOP A ONE-NAP ROUTINE. Once you are ready to make the switch to one nap a day, it's very helpful to associate the afternoon nap with lunch. That is, have naptime follow lunchtime every day. Regina did this with her son Anthony. Every day, Regina gave Anthony his lunch at 12:00. After lunch, she cleaned him up, took him to her bedroom, read him a favorite story, closed the shades, and put him in his crib for his nap. On days that Anthony woke up earlier than usual or seemed especially tired, she would move lunch earlier, even to 10:30 or 11:00. This way she could put him down for a nap earlier, but still make sure that the nap-after-lunch routine was always followed.

Transitioning to No Nap

Sometime between three and four, most children give up taking a nap. Many children, however, continue to take a nap until the age of five, or even six. The following figure shows the percentage of children who nap at different ages.

WHAT ARE THE SIGNS? The most common sign that your child is ready to stop napping is that he will simply stop falling asleep at naptime. Another sign is that he'll take a much longer time to fall asleep. A third sign is that on days that he misses his nap, he does fine. On days that your child does not nap, if he does not appear tired and does not become cranky or irritable, it is likely that he is ready to give up his nap.

DON'T GIVE UP ON NAPS TOO QUICKLY. Often parents think that if their child hasn't fallen asleep at naptime for a few days, their child has given up naps. It doesn't happen this way. Naps are typically not given up so quickly. Just because your child doesn't take a nap for a few days in a row doesn't mean that he is ready to

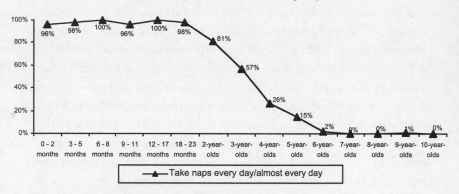

Percentage of Children Taking Naps

— Take naps every day/almost every day

Source: 2004 National Sleep Foundation *Sleep in America* poll

give them up altogether. Stick with your usual nap routine for at least another few weeks and see what happens.

HOW TO MAKE THE TRANSITION. Just like the transition from two naps to one afternoon nap, the transition to no naps will likely not happen all at once. Your child may need a nap on some days and not on others. He may go through a period of not needing a nap, and then suddenly return to napping for a while—perhaps the result of starting preschool or other activities or changes that tire him out.

INSTITUTE QUIET TIME. Even if your child doesn't need to sleep in the afternoon, establish quiet time or rest time instead. This will give everyone a chance to recharge, and it will give your child the opportunity to fall asleep if needed. It is recommended that quiet time occur in your child's room. Feel free to let her bring toys or books into bed. Some parents, however, choose to have a quiet time of watching a video in the living room or family room.

Naps are good not only for your baby but also for you if you are at home with your child. They are often a great mental and physical restorative: you can have a few minutes of peace and quiet to play with your other children, do some household chores, call a friend, watch your favorite soap opera, or take a nap yourself. When your child is ready to give up naps, quiet time can offer the same benefits to parents and children. Katie's mother had her daughter have quiet time in a playpen in the living room rather than putting her in her crib in the bedroom. Katie had lots of toys to play with and learned that this was quiet time. To help with the transition to quiet time, Katie was put in her playpen for progressively longer times, beginning with five minutes and working up to forty-five minutes. Katie's mother enjoyed the peace and quiet, and Katie learned to play by herself. This concept of learning to play alone is an important skill that your child needs to acquire. Your child needs to learn how to entertain herself and be on her own. This will be important as she gets older, especially when she starts school and is required to work on her own.

MOVE BEDTIME EARLIER. Once your child has given up his daytime nap, you will likely need to move bedtime earlier. Your little one may be exhausted earlier in the evening. An earlier bedtime will help ensure that he gets the sleep that he needs.

WHAT TO DO IF YOUR CHILD STILL NAPS BUT WON'T FALL ASLEEP AT BEDTIME. Often, between the ages of three and four, young children go through a period in which they clearly still need their afternoon nap but it interferes with their ability to fall asleep at bedtime. This phase can last several months. You can deal with it by moving your child's bedtime later by an hour or so, until she is ready to give up naps. Another option is to keep bedtime the same, but let your child "read" books or play quietly in bed for another hour or so. Leandra did this with Christopher, age three and a half. For several months, she stuck with his usual 7:30 bedtime but set a timer for forty-five minutes during which Christopher could play in his bed with some toys. When the timer went off, his toys got put away and the bedroom light was turned off. If he called out to his parents during this extra playtime, the light was turned off early. It worked perfectly. Christopher would happily play quietly in his room, Leandra got to stick with their usual family evening routine, and Christopher fell asleep quickly when the lights were turned off.

NAPTIME PROBLEMS

It can be incredibly frustrating to have a baby who doesn't nap during the day. In fact, parents are often more frustrated by naptime problems than they are by nighttime problems. Not only does the baby get cranky, but so do the parents.

If you are having naptime problems as well as bedtime-nighttime problems, you have several choices. First, you or your caregiver can do what you normally do: rock your child to sleep, feed him, or drive him in the car. Another choice is to do the same checking method at naptime as you do at bedtime. It may not be advisable to do this simultaneously with the basic bedtime method (see page 100). It may be too much for you and your baby. Wait until your child gets the hang of falling asleep independently at bedtime. Then do sleep training at naptime. The ultimate goal is to have your child falling asleep in the same manner and sleeping in the same place at all naptimes, at bedtime, and throughout the night.

The best plan of action if you are having naptime, bedtime, and/or night-waking problems is to solve things one step at a time in the following order:

1. Bedtime
2. Wait two weeks
3. Nighttime
4. Wait two weeks
5. Naptime

THE BASIC NAPTIME METHOD

The basic naptime method is based on the notion discussed in Chapter 6 of replacing your baby's negative sleep associations with positive sleep associations. A step-by-step guide is provided here to help you through this process.

- ✦ **Before starting: Solve bedtime and nighttime issues.** Before starting to solve naptime issues, be sure that your child is able to fall asleep on his own at bedtime and is sleeping through the night. If you rock your child to sleep at bedtime, and he sleeps through the night after that point but doesn't nap well during the day, you first need to make changes at bedtime. What happens regarding sleep at night will definitely affect sleep at other times.

- ✦ **Step one: Naptime schedule.** Step one is to have a set time, or times, for your baby to take a nap. Your baby needs to nap at the same time every day, once she is past nine to twelve months. Before that age, you can use the *two-hour rule* method discussed earlier. If you put your baby or toddler down to nap at exactly the same time every day, it will help set his internal clock so that his body becomes attuned to falling asleep at exactly that time. Be sure not to wait too long to put your child down for a nap, or you will miss your window of opportunity. Hit the right moment and he'll fall asleep quickly. Wait too long and he'll be overtired, making it much harder for him to settle down.

- ✦ **Step two: Mini naptime routine.** Step two is to establish a consistent naptime routine. Just as with a bedtime routine, a naptime routine is essential to your child's being able to fall asleep easily and quickly. It helps your child calm down and get ready for the transition from being awake to falling asleep. This should be a mini version of your bedtime routine. Obviously, you won't give your child a bath or change into pajamas, but you can definitely sing the same song or read the same two books. Also, just as with your bedtime routine, the naptime routine should be done in your child's room so that there is an easy transition from the routine to bed. Similarly, reading, cuddling, and singing should end before your child falls asleep.

✦ **Step three: Put down awake.** Yes, again, this is the hard part. Your child needs to learn to fall asleep on his own at naptime. After your child's naptime routine is done, put him in his crib or bed, say night-night, and leave the room. Your child will probably call for you, cry, or scream. Wait. Then do a simple checking routine. Go back into your child's room. Tell him that it is okay. Tell him again that it is time for him to go to sleep. Don't pick him up. Don't cuddle him. Be gentle but firm. Remain fairly neutral and stay for a brief time, no more than one minute. Make the visits brief and boring. Leave. Wait again. Check again. Repeatedly wait and then check on your child if he is upset or calls for you.

How long should you wait before checking on your child? Check on your child as frequently or infrequently as you wish. As with the bedtime method (see Chapter 6), how often you check on your child entirely depends on your tolerance level and your child's temperament. Some parents can't bear to listen to their child cry for more than thirty seconds. That is okay. Wait only thirty seconds before checking. The longer you can wait, the better, but it doesn't really matter. Some children, however, get more upset when they see their parents. If this is the case, wait longer periods rather than shorter ones. Check on your child, though, rather than letting him cry it out until he falls asleep. Not checking seems to prolong the process. Remember, the goal is to have your child fall asleep on his own, not to make your child upset. All that you want is that golden moment when your child falls asleep independently.

HOW LONG SHOULD YOU CONTINUE? Naptime training is much harder than doing sleep training at bedtime. At bedtime, your child is more tired (what some experts call "sleep pressure"), and there is a whole night ahead. With naps, there is not as much need for sleep, and there is still an entire day ahead. Give it either thirty minutes or sixty minutes. At the end of that time, go get your child, announcing, "Oh, you must not be tired," and go on with your day. If your child usually takes another nap later in the day, keep him up until then, or keep him awake until bedtime (playing with water, whether in the sink or in a bathtub, invariably keeps even the sleepiest baby awake). You can also take a fifteen- to thirty-minute break and try again. Whatever you do, don't let your child fall asleep elsewhere, or while nursing or lying down with you. If your child starts falling asleep, even ten minutes later, announce again, "Oh, you must be tired," and take him back to his crib.

DOING IT ONE STEP AT A TIME. Rather than do a crash course in naptime training, it is sometimes better to take it one step at a time. As a start, take a week or two simply to establish a schedule. Decide when your child is going to nap and set her schedule. For example, when Teesha's daughter, Amber, was seven months old, Teesha took her out for a car ride at 9:30 and 2:30 every day for a week. Within a week, Amber's internal clock was set and she was falling asleep quickly in the car. For the next week, Teesha added a naptime routine of reading the same story in her daughter's room each naptime before putting her in the car. Finally, in the third week, she started naptime training, for only the first nap. She chose the morning nap because that was when Amber fell asleep most quickly. To make sure that Amber didn't become so sleep deprived that it would interfere with her nighttime sleep, Teesha continued to go for her usual afternoon car ride for Amber's second nap. In the fourth week, she moved all naps to Amber's crib. By taking it one step at a time, she was able to solve Teesha's naptime problems.

WHAT TO DO IF YOUR CHILD NAPS FOR ONLY THIRTY MINUTES BUT CLEARLY NEEDS MORE. At first, many babies undergoing sleep training will take only a short nap, waking up cranky and irritable after just thirty or forty-five minutes, whereas if they had been rocked to sleep or put in the swing, they would have slept for an hour or two. Think of this as a normal nighttime awakening. It is a normal arousal, and your baby likely can't fall back to sleep on his own. As your baby gets better and better at self-soothing to sleep at naptime, his naps will naturally start getting longer because he'll be able to fall right back to sleep on his own. In the meantime, you can try holding him or giving him his pacifier or whatever he needs to get him to sleep longer, just as when handling night wakings during sleep training at bedtime.

Rarely is it effective to leave your baby to cry in hopes that he'll fall back to sleep. It just doesn't seem to work. Your baby has slept just enough to take the edge off of his sleepiness, making it hard for him to fall back to sleep on his own. So go get your baby and see if you can help him go back to sleep. If not, then wait until the next naptime or bedtime. As your baby learns to self-soothe, this problem will likely resolve on its own.

WHAT TO DO IF YOUR CHILD NAPS WELL AT CHILD CARE BUT NOT AT HOME. Often infants and toddlers nap well at child care but refuse to nap at home. If this is the case, speak to your child care provider. Find out what is going on at child care that works so well and duplicate it at home. This is also a sign that your child really does need to nap and can do it, giving you the resolve to make some changes at home. If the opposite is true—your child naps great at home but not at child care—again compare notes and see if your child care provider can duplicate what's working at home.

Reminders ————————————————————————

- ✦ There are no absolute rules about naps, but there are guidelines as to how many times a day your baby should nap and for how long.
- ✦ Most toddlers transition to one nap a day by eighteen months.
- ✦ Most children stop taking naps between three and four years of age.
- ✦ Scheduling problems and negative sleep associations are the primary reasons that children have naptime problems.
- ✦ Use the basic naptime method to solve nap problems. First, though, resolve bedtime and then nighttime issues.

CHAPTER 8

What About Cosleeping?:
Making the Choice and Making the Transition

Ruth has always loved having her children sleep with her. From the day she brought each home from the hospital, she has had them sleep in bed with her and her husband. She finds it much easier to breast-feed with the baby in bed with her. She's never even bought a crib, as she has always known that sleeping together as a family is important to her.

Consuela always assumed that she would have her baby sleep with her, just as the rest of her family has always had their babies sleep with them. However, she has found cosleeping very difficult. She worries all night long that she is going to roll over onto the baby, and every time the baby moves, Consuela wakes up. She feels as though she hasn't gotten any sleep since the baby was born. Although the baby is only four months old, Consuela would like to make a change.

Diane and Phil enjoy having their ten-month-old and three-year-old boys come join them in bed at 5:00 each morning. They call this special time of the day their "snuggle bug time."

Janet and Larry have three children. Throughout the night, they play "musical beds," with no one seeming to end up in the right bed. The baby usually ends up sleeping in his swing. Janet usually ends up sleeping in their bed with their five-year-old, and Larry often ends up in the guest room bed.

SHARING A ROOM WITH YOUR BABY

In the first few weeks after their baby's birth, many parents keep their babies in their bedroom, often in a bassinet or crib within arm's reach. Those first few weeks are often a blur, with little distinction between day and night. It all seems to be a long series of feedings, burpings, and diaper changes with a few stolen moments of sleep thrown in. After the constant need for frequent feedings abates, which can happen in anywhere from two weeks to three months, you will want to consider whether or not to move your baby to her own room. Of course, this will be the case only if you have a choice. Parents who live in one-bedroom apartments or who reside with other family members may not have this option.

There are both advantages and disadvantages to having your baby as a roommate. The advantages include continued ease in responding to your baby in the middle of the night. When your baby wants to feed or gets fussy, you won't have to go as far to soothe her. Some parents also find it very nice to be able to look over during the night to check on their baby and just enjoy her presence.

One of the major disadvantages of having your baby as a roommate is that it results in less sleep for everyone. The parents get less sleep because every time the baby whimpers there is the temptation to respond to her. How can you not, when she is within arm's reach? You are also likely to awaken more frequently just to check on her. Babies also get less sleep when they sleep in their parents' bedroom. Many studies have shown that most babies who share a room with their parents do not sleep through the night. This is probably because you are more likely to pick her up when she fusses, which results in less sleep for her, too. Also, your activities during the night are going to keep her up, just as hers will keep you up.

Another disadvantage is the difficulty in eventually moving the baby to her own room. The longer you wait, the harder it will be.

The baby will get used to sharing a room with her parents and will find it difficult to make the transition to being on her own as she becomes older. While a two- to three-week-old baby will not know the difference, a six-month-old will.

No matter what you hear and read, though, you need to do what feels right for you. If it feels right to share your room with your baby, then do so. If it doesn't, don't.

SHARING A BED WITH YOUR BABY

Even if you have your baby in your room, you may or may not be sharing your bed with him. Some parents prefer cosleeping, and there are several groups who believe that it is more natural than our society's typical practice of having babies sleep alone in their own rooms. Again, do what is right for you.

As with sharing a room, there are a number of positive and negative aspects to cosleeping. Some of the positives, in addition to those mentioned above, include:

- ✦ Some believe that cosleeping is essential to a child's emotional development. Some argue that it is more "natural," as indicated by the high level of cosleeping in many societies.
- ✦ Sharing a bed can give you extra time with your baby, especially if you work during the day.
- ✦ Some research shows that babies who cosleep may be at less risk for SIDS than babies who sleep alone. The key may be that babies who cosleep keep their breathing in tune with their mothers'. Other studies, however, report an increased risk of SIDS. At this time, it is not clear whether sharing a bed with your baby increases or decreases the risk of SIDS.

There are also several drawbacks to cosleeping:

✦ Babies who share a bed with their parents tend to have sleep problems. They will have difficulties falling asleep at night without their parents' presence and will wake frequently during the night. This is because babies who share a bed with their parents do not learn how to fall asleep on their own, an integral part of sleeping through the night.

✦ Another drawback is deciding when cosleeping should stop. At what age do you decide that your child needs to sleep on his own in his own room? Again, similar to sharing a room, the longer you wait, the more difficult the transition may be for your baby.

✦ Safety is another concern. Although it is very unlikely that you will roll over and harm your baby, babies can be smothered by pillows and comforters or fall between the bed and the wall.

✦ If your baby can fall asleep only when sharing a bed with you, you are going to have problems leaving your baby with a babysitter, a grandparent, or anyone else.

✦ Another drawback is the potential effect on your marriage or relationship. It is difficult to have an adult or private conversation when a child is sleeping in the same bed. And it is deadly to your sex life. Parents worry enough that their lovemaking will wake a child who is in the next room. When sharing a room with a child, it is much more of a concern. And when the baby is in the same bed, the possibility of spontaneous lovemaking goes out the window. This may be okay with one of you, but it can also cause tension between you and your partner.

Finally, it is important to decide whether having the baby sleeping in bed with you is for the baby's sake or for your own sake. If you are a single parent or your partner is frequently out of town overnight or works the night shift, you may be continuing the cosleeping because it is nice to have a warm, cuddly body in bed with you. On the other hand, some people encourage cosleeping as a way to keep a barrier between themselves and their bed partner. If one of you is not interested in sex, having a baby in bed with you will keep the focus off this issue. If this is the case, it is important to communicate with your partner and not use the baby to avoid dealing with your problems. Be sure that the cosleeping is not a way to avoid facing other issues and that it is not being done to fulfill needs you have that should be met by other means.

DIFFERENT KINDS OF COSLEEPING

As depicted by the families at the beginning of the chapter, there are many reasons why children sleep in their parents' bed, and many different arrangements. Basically, though, there are two types of cosleeping: lifestyle choice and reactive cosleeping.

Lifestyle Choice

Cosleeping may be a lifestyle choice in which parents decide that they want to share their bed (or bedroom) with their baby. Sometimes this is referred to as sleep sharing or having a family bed. Marissa made this decision with each of her two children. When the baby arrived home from the hospital, she began having the baby sleep in bed with her. She thought that it was important to have the baby close to her throughout the night, and that it helped with bonding. She kept each child in bed with her until two years of age. At that point, she transitioned them to their own bedroom. Lucinda also chose to share her bed with her toddler, but just in the morning. When Evan woke up in the morning, it was a family tradition for him to come snuggle in bed with his parents. They all loved their morning cuddle time and sometimes everyone got another hour or two of sleep.

Reactive Cosleeping

In reactive cosleeping, the baby or toddler ends up in the parents' bed at night, but it's not totally by choice; rather, it's a way to solve a sleep problem. Parents sometimes find it easier to bring their child into bed with them when their child resists falling asleep in the crib or wakes up several times during the night. They may not like it very much, but they haven't found a better solution or are too exhausted to fight the battle.

Cathy was struggling with having her baby in her bed. Emily woke up several times a night. The first few times each night, Cathy would nurse her back to sleep, but usually by 4:00 a.m. she was so tired of getting up that she just brought Emily to her bed, though she really wished that Emily would sleep through the night in her crib.

Thomas and Tina faced the same issue with their three-year-old, Dylan. They would often find Dylan in their bed in the morning. If either one woke up when Dylan came in during the night, they would return him to his own room. However, Dylan had figured out that if he climbed in on his father's side of the bed rather than his mother's side, then his parents usually slept through his arrival.

MAKING THE CHOICE

Whether you decide to share a room and/or a bed with your baby is a family decision. It is a personal choice and there is no absolute right or wrong decision. Talk it over with your partner (if you have one) and decide what works best for your family. Try not to be swayed by what others say.

If you decide that you want to cosleep for a while, but that you want your baby sleeping in his own crib in the long run, it's best to make the transition to the crib by three months of age. After three months, habits are fairly ingrained and it will be harder on your baby (and you) to make the change. So try envisioning where you would like your baby sleeping when he is a year old. If you want him with you, then there is no need to do anything. If you want him sleeping in a crib in his own room, then try to make the change by three months. Obviously, this doesn't mean that you cannot make the change at a later age, such as at nine months, but realize that it will likely be more difficult for everyone.

COMBINING SOLITARY SLEEPING AND COSLEEPING

You may not have one exclusive sleeping arrangement in your household. For example, your baby may fall asleep in his crib but join you when he wakes at night. Or your toddler may fall asleep in your bed but then be moved to his own bed when you are ready to go to bed for the night. Or an early-morning cuddle with everyone in the bed may be the choice that you make. Realize that cosleeping is not an either-or decision. There are lots of gradations in between.

MAKING COSLEEPING WORK

If you choose to have your baby sleep with you in your bed or bedroom, there are several considerations to make it work.

+ **Safety.** Safety should be the top concern of all parents who have a child share their bed. See the information

Cosleeping Safety

Be sure to keep your baby safe if she sleeps in bed with you.

+ Use a firm mattress and avoid using heavy blankets and comforters. Pillows can also be a suffocation risk.
+ Don't sleep with your baby on a sofa, chair, or waterbed.
+ Be sure that your baby can't roll off the sides or end of the bed and can't get trapped between the mattress and the wall. Check that the mattress fits tightly against the headboard.
+ Make sure that your baby does not get too warm.
+ Don't let infants and toddlers sleep next to each other.
+ Don't let pets share a bed with you and your baby.
+ Don't sleep with your baby if you or your bed partner has a sleep disorder, such as sleep apnea.
+ Don't sleep with your baby if you or your bed partner drinks alcohol or takes any other type of drugs or medication that makes you sleepy.
+ Don't sleep with your baby if you are ill or are unusually tired.

in the box provided above on keeping your child safe when sleeping in bed with you. Other ways to keep your baby safe are to use a side car or a cosleeper which is like a bassinet that attaches to the side of the bed. This gives a baby a safe place to sleep while being right next to the parents.

+ **Make sure everyone agrees.** If there is going to be more than one parent who will be sharing the bed with the baby, make sure that everyone agrees with the arrangement. In order for cosleeping to be a family choice, all family members must agree to it. This can be a difficult

conversation, but it's an important one for the relationship of the parents.

✦ **Make sure everyone gets enough sleep.** When babies
sleep with their parents, they usually need their parents
present to fall asleep. This usually means that the parents have to go to bed when the baby goes to bed.
Parents are often not ready to go to bed at 7:00 or 8:00 in
the evening and thus keep the baby up later, such as until 9:00 or 9:30. If you are going to have your baby sleep
with you, you need to make compromises so that you are
on your baby's schedule, rather than putting your baby
on your schedule.

WHEN TO MOVE A CHILD OUT OF YOUR BED

There is no prescribed right time to move a child out of your bed or
bedroom. There is also no age by which you must make the change,
although making the switch by three months is easiest on your baby
if you want your baby sleeping in her own crib for the long run. A
child does not have to be in her own bed by age three, four, or even
five years. Make the change when you and your child are ready. This
will be at a different time for every family. It may even occur at different ages for different children within the same family. Some families wait until their child indicates that she wants to sleep in her
own room, although not all children come to this conclusion.

Don't make the transition, however, when there are other
changes going on, such as when beginning toilet training or starting
preschool. It's too much for a child to deal with more than one
change at a time. Instead, wait until things have settled down again.
When you do start, make a few small changes at a time, as outlined
below, and make the move gradually.

MAKING THE TRANSITION FROM COSLEEPING

The transition from cosleeping to having your child sleep in her own crib or bed can occur at three months, at a year, or not until three years. The older the child, the longer the transition may take. Remember, this is going to be a major change for your child, so you should expect a few bumps along the way. As with the basic bedtime method outlined on page 100, you can start by making changes only at bedtime, continuing to bring your child into bed with you during naptime. Also, if your child doesn't already have a favorite comfort object, such as a stuffed animal, a doll, or a blanket, try encouraging her to start using one (see more information on transitional objects in Chapter 5). Having a lovey nearby will make the transition easier.

There are many possible points where you can start making this transition, such as at bedtime as discussed above. Where to start will depend on your child's tolerance to change and how quickly you want to make the transition. Here are some potential places to start.

+ **Naptime.** If your child is still taking naps during the day, you can start having him nap in his own room. Some parents choose to make the change first at naptime rather than at bedtime, especially if evenings are chaotic in their household.

+ **Bedtime routine.** Another good place to start is to begin doing your child's bedtime routine in his room (see Chapter 5 for more information on bedtime routines). Change into pajamas, sing a song, and read books (or do whatever you do as part of your child's usual bedtime routine) in his room. At the end of the routine, bring him to your bed to fall asleep.

+ **Sleeping on the parents' bedroom floor.** Another way to make a gradual change is to make your child his own special bed on your bedroom floor. This bed can be a sleeping bag, a futon, or an extra mattress. Put it at the foot of your bed or someplace in your room. This will allow your child to feel the security of being near you while getting used to sleeping independently. Obviously, this is a choice only if your child is a toddler or older.

✦ **Move yourself into your child's room.** Another alternative is to move both of you into your child's room until your child adjusts to sleeping there. Once he's comfortable and sleeping well, then you can gradually move yourself out. Go from lying down with him to sitting next to him as he falls asleep, then from sitting on the bed to sitting on the floor, and finally move from being near the bed to his doorway.

✦ **Falling asleep independently.** The key to your child sleeping in his own room all night is having him fall asleep independently at bedtime. You can take this in one giant step by tucking him in when he is still awake at bedtime and leaving the room. If you take this one giant step, be sure and check on your child until he is asleep. See Chapter 6 on doing the basic bedtime method to help your child fall asleep independently and learn to self-soothe to sleep.

✦ **During the night.** As you work on helping your child fall asleep independently, continue to go to your child throughout the night when he wakes up. At first you may want to bring him to your bed or stay with him until he returns to sleep. Before making any major changes in what you do during the night, however, wait until your child is falling asleep easily and quickly at bedtime for at least two weeks. At that point, he is likely to start sleeping naturally for longer stretches as he develops the skill of being able to put himself back to sleep when he awakens during the night. At some point, however, you may need to make some changes during the night as well, such as checking on your child during the night rather than bringing him to your bed.

WHAT TO DO IF YOUR TODDLER RESISTS THE MOVE. Expect some difficulties at bedtime and some late-night visits from an older child. You need to decide how to handle these. Some families keep an extra mattress on their bedroom floor for those middle-of-the-night visits. Other families simply snuggle in with their child when their child awakens. And other families decide that once the move is made there is no going back, and their child must sleep in his own bed. If it is important to you that your child sleep in his own room throughout the night, then calmly and gently lead him back to bed throughout the night, or check on him and let him know that it is night-night time and you'll see him in the morning.

As your child is going through this transition, reward him for his accomplishments. This is especially the case for an older child. Praise him and give him lots of encouragement for his successes, such as falling asleep in his new bed with you there or sleeping in his own bed all night (even if there were lots of middle-of-the-night visits).

Reminders

+ There are many reasons why families share a bedroom or a bed with their child.
+ Sharing a bed with your baby has advantages and disadvantages.
+ Parents who sleep with their baby may do so as a family lifestyle choice or as a response to a sleep problem.
+ Make a decision regarding cosleeping that is right for your family.
+ Ensure that your baby is safe when cosleeping.
+ Make the transition from cosleeping to solitary sleeping in gradual steps.

PART THREE

Steps for Success

CHAPTER 9

"Am I Doing the Right Thing?": How to Cope with Sleep Training

Michelle and Tom's sixteen-month-old son, Sean, had never slept through the night. Every night either Michelle or Tom would rock Sean to sleep while he drank from a bottle. On the first night of sleep training, Michelle put Sean in his crib awake after reading him a story and singing him a song. After listening to Sean cry for ten minutes, Michelle herself started crying. Both Michelle and Tom felt guilty doing nothing, listening to Sean cry when he seemed to really need them. They kept reading over and over again what they were supposed to do, reassuring each other that they were doing the right thing. Eventually Sean fell asleep, and within three days he was falling asleep quickly at bedtime and was sleeping through the night.

A difficult issue that many parents face is how to cope with a screaming baby. It's very hard when your two-year-old has been sobbing for Mommy or Daddy for forty-five minutes, and you know that if you just rocked him for five minutes, he would calm down and immediately fall asleep. This is where the going gets tough and why parents often do not succeed in making the necessary changes to help their child sleep through the night.

GUILT

One thing that seems to go hand in hand with being a parent is guilt. Am I doing enough for my baby? Am I a good parent? These are difficult questions in themselves without also having to cope with setting limits and possibly upsetting your child at times.

Unfortunately, setting limits for your child is part of being a good parent. Children are born as clean slates. They don't know anything, which is an overwhelming concept to realize. This means that you have to teach them everything. You have to teach them to feed themselves, to dress themselves, how to do laundry, and even how to calculate the tip at a restaurant. You have to teach them to distinguish between right and wrong. As part of that, you have to teach them how to behave. For example, you don't hit people. You don't jump up and down screaming in church or synagogue. You don't scratch yourself in certain places in public. And on and on. It's a tough job, so don't feel too guilty when your child doesn't like what you just told him to do. It comes with the territory of being a parent.

Many working parents worry that they are not spending enough time with their children if they put them to bed shortly after getting home from work. Ken was worried that he wasn't spending any quality time with his fifteen-month-old, Justin. Ken got home from work each night at 7:00, just when Justin was getting ready to go to bed. Stacey had the same concern, but with an added issue: she wondered whether it was fair to her three-year-old, Joshua, to put him to bed early without spending any time with her after having been in day care all day. She felt that it was just another instance when Joshua got pushed aside and didn't get to spend time with her.

These parents' concerns are very real and very common. But keep in mind that it is just as important for your child to get adequate sleep at night. Numerous studies have shown the negative consequences of sleep deprivation and the positive effects of sleep on development. Proper sleep not only will put your child in better spirits but will allow him to learn more and enjoy the time that he does spend with you. It is important that your child have adequate time with you, but these times can be early in the morning or on your days off. He will be at a disadvantage, though, if he doesn't get adequate sleep—even if it is just for one night.

QUESTIONS PARENTS OFTEN ASK

Here are some of the questions parents frequently ask about sleep training.

"AM I A BAD PARENT?" A bad parent is someone who doesn't provide for her child or abuses her child. A good parent is someone who takes care of her children's needs and does the right thing. Teaching your child how to fall asleep on his own is doing the right thing. Part of being a good parent is doing the hard stuff, and that can include teaching your child how to fall asleep independently. Many of us want to be the "nice" parent, but that's not always being the "good" parent.

"WILL THIS CAUSE MY CHILD HARM?" As long as you provide your baby with lots of attention during the day, you will not harm your child by letting her cry at bedtime. Some say that sleep training simply gives parents permission to allow their baby to cry. This is not exactly true. One aspect of dealing with sleep problems may involve your baby crying, but that is not the largest component. The major components are teaching your child how to be a self-soother and how to put herself to sleep. Prevention of sleep problems is even more important. By preventing future problems, you are helping your child, not harming her.

"WILL THIS AFFECT MY CHILD'S ATTACHMENT TO ME?" There has been a great deal of research over the past decade on the importance of infant-parent attachment. A few studies have assessed the impact of sleep training on attachment. These studies have actually found that young children are more securely attached to their parents following sleep training.

"WILL MY CHILD BE EMOTIONALLY SCARRED FOR LIFE?" Some parents envision their child on the psychiatrist's couch talking about the damage his parents did to him by letting him cry at bedtime. This will not happen. Research has shown that children who sleep well, with limited bedtime problems and night-waking problems, are better adjusted and better behaved, and do better overall. One study done in our laboratory found that those children between the ages of two and three who had bedtime problems were more likely to have a whole spectrum of behavior or psychological problems. That is, they were more likely to be aggressive and noncompliant. They were also more likely to appear depressed and withdrawn. Other recent studies of longer-term outcomes and the benefits of sleeping well are under way. For example, one study found a relationship between sleep problems in toddlers and preschoolers with later behavior problems in middle school. So rather than scarring your child by sleep training, you will be helping him. Children who sleep well are well-adjusted and have fewer overall problems.

"WILL MY CHILD STILL LOVE ME IN THE MORNING?" Don't worry; your child will still love you in the morning. He is not upset with you personally when he is crying at night; he simply wants to fall asleep. The next morning he will be just as happy to see you as always.

THE EMOTIONAL ASPECTS OF SLEEP

For some reason, we seem to attach much more emotional weight to sleep than to practically any other aspect of our children's lives. There are probably many reasons for this. A few of these reasons will be explored here. It is important to understand these reasons so that they can be dealt with in a forthright manner and not interfere with what you decide is best for your child.

We all have long-standing images of an adorable sleeping baby. Some of our favorite pictures are of our child asleep. In sleep, babies seem sweet and vulnerable. When dreaming of having one's own child, many people have the image of cuddling a baby to sleep in a rocking chair in a peaceful, quiet place. So when your child is sobbing at bedtime, it runs counter to these pleasant images of cuddling together.

Second, we tend to give dramatic meanings to the cries of a baby alone in a crib. With older children we learn why they are upset because they can tell us. With young babies, however, we really don't know why they are crying and often attribute their cries to hunger, sadness, separation anxiety, or any number of concerns. Rather than simply thinking that the baby is saying, "I don't want to be here. Take me out of my crib," we believe our child is saying something completely different, such as, "You have abandoned me." Thus, we often interpret our baby's cries as separation anxiety or abandonment, which may not be the case at all.

We also don't like to think about our children being sad and alone. The picture of our child crying all alone in his crib evokes an almost irresistible need to comfort our child. It is difficult to stand by and let this happen even when we know that it is best for the child.

Be careful not to project too many of your own feelings onto your baby when he is crying. Your baby does not hate you, and you are not abandoning him. You are trying to do what is best for him, and that includes finding a way for both of you to get a good night's sleep. Your baby needs you. He needs you to help him learn how to fall asleep on his own.

It may be helpful to remind yourself that falling asleep alone is a skill that has to be learned, akin to learning to walk. When he is learning to walk, he will probably fall down a few times. This may scare him and make him cry. Being scared and crying doesn't mean, however, that you will never let him try to walk alone. That would be harmful. Try to see sleep the same way. Your baby may be upset at first, but eventually, with some practice, your baby will acquire this new skill and have it for a lifetime.

―――

Bedtime had always been a struggle. Vanessa decided that she needed to replace a stressful bedtime routine with a calm one that would help her daughter, Denise, go to sleep happy and relaxed. Once she developed a set bedtime routine to help Denise fall asleep on her own, home life changed dramatically. There were no more crying spells when Vanessa announced it was bedtime, and Denise seemed much happier in the evenings and during the day. Three weeks after beginning the routine, Vanessa received a wonderful surprise. Dinner was over, and she was reading Denise a story in the living room. Halfway through the story, Denise turned toward her mother, lifted her arms, and said, "Bed." Thinking that she had misheard, Vanessa asked Denise to repeat what she had said. In a more definite tone, Denise announced that it was time for bed.

―――

Your child may not go to this extreme, but she will stop dreading bedtime and enjoy the peacefulness of crawling into a snug bed after a busy day.

PARENTS WITH TWO DIFFERENT STYLES

Some couples work well together dealing with their child's sleep problems. As one mother said, "We had a common enemy." For others, sleep problems may cause disagreements. One parent may be willing to let the baby cry, while the other may not be able to tolerate it. One may not like having the baby share their bed, while the other may not mind. Leslie and Mark were such a couple.

Leslie and Mark's son, Danny, woke several times a night, always needing to be rocked to sleep. By the time Danny was seven months old, Leslie decided that it was time to do something. She couldn't take the sleepless nights much longer. One Thursday night, she put Danny down in his crib awake rather than rocking him to sleep. After five minutes of listening to Danny cry, Mark stormed upstairs to get Danny, saying that he couldn't take it. This led to several weeks of arguing over what they should do. Both thought that something should be done, but while Leslie could tolerate Danny being upset, it was too difficult for Mark.

How can this issue be resolved? Communicate. Compromise. Negotiate. Marriage can be difficult even in the best of times. And when we are sleep deprived, even the best of us get cranky. In developing a strategy, both individuals need to have input; otherwise, sleep training will not work. Both people have to come to an agreement. This will require communication on both sides. Don't simply agree for the sake of avoiding an argument—the process will backfire. One of you will end up insisting on a different course of action in the middle of dealing with your baby at bedtime. That course of action is usually to give up and get the baby when he is upset. This will make the situation worse, especially if the baby has been crying for a long time. It will teach your baby that if he persists and really screams, someone will come to get him. You have just taught him to cry longer and louder. The next time that you try to implement sleep training, your baby will be upset twice as long. Therefore, for the sake of you, your partner, and your child, it is vital that you discuss what you are going to do, develop a strategy, and stick to it. This process will be good practice: developing a strategy to deal with your child's sleep problems will be just the first of many times that you will need to negotiate solutions to a child-rearing problem, whether it is because your child bites, is acting up in school, or keeps breaking his curfew.

There is another practical way to deal with two parents who have different styles. Often one parent can deal with sleep training while the other parent can't. If this is the case in your family, allow the parent who can cope best to do the sleep training the first night or two. Plan to do it when the one who can't cope is out of town or at least out of the house. He or she can go to the movies, visit a friend for an evening or two, go for a long walk, or listen to music with headphones on. After the first night or two, that parent can rejoin the bedtime routine.

One other hint: It is important that each parent put the child to sleep on different nights. If not, your child may not be able to fall asleep for the other parent.

HOW TO COPE

You will probably need a repertoire of strategies for coping with a crying baby at bedtime because one method will not work in every situation. Here are some suggestions that many parents have found helpful.

DAMPEN THE NOISE. The sound of your baby's crying is likely to make you feel stressed. That is nature's way of making sure that babies are taken care of. Unfortunately, the sound of your baby's crying will raise your level of stress whether it is an emergency situation or your baby is simply fussy or unhappy. One way to decrease your response is to dampen the noise. Don't block out all the noise, since you do want to make sure that you don't ignore a baby who is in danger. But if you know that your baby is simply unhappy and likely to be crying for a while, then dampen the noise. Go to another part of the house. Turn on a fan or the air vent in your kitchen. Turn on the vacuum cleaner. Take a shower or simply sit in the bathroom with the shower or sink faucet running. Put some music on or turn up the television. Blow-dry your hair.

Many parents worry that these noises will keep the baby awake. Don't worry; as long as you're not making too much noise, any constant sound is likely to help your baby sleep. It is also much less likely to keep your baby awake than hearing you wandering around the house.

DON'T BE A CLOCK WATCHER. Remember the old saying "A watched pot never boils"? This is true about babies also. A watched baby will seem never to stop crying. When your child is crying, don't watch the clock. This will make the crying seem to go on forever. Don't sit on the stairs listening. Go somewhere else in the house. Do something else. Put the dishes in the dishwasher. Flip through a magazine. Put on your favorite music. Call a friend for support while your child is crying (and be sure to explain what is going on!). Go get the mail from the mailbox. Do anything but watch the clock.

HUMOR YOURSELF. One of the best ways to deal with a stressful situation is to use humor. Humor is a great stress reducer, and it will help you keep your perspective. When it is 10:00 at night and your baby has been cranky all day and you are now on your eleventh trip to check on your crying baby, it is easy to lose all perspective. You will feel as though you will never have a moment's peace again. But try to remember that this is just a temporary situation. As your grandmother probably once told you, "this, too, shall pass."

So use humor to keep your sanity. Cut out cartoons about babies who don't sleep and put them on the refrigerator. Look at them to remind yourself that you are not alone. Put notes up around the house. Put a sign on the door to your baby's room saying CRYING BABY—ENTER AT YOUR OWN RISK. Put a sign for visitors in a prominent place: WE ARE TEACHING SAM TO SLEEP THROUGH THE NIGHT. EXPECT DIRTY DISHES, CRYING BABIES, AND UNHAPPY PARENTS. PLEASE PROVIDE SUPPORT.

SMILE. Smiling is the best thing to do when you are feeling low. You cannot feel stressed or be unhappy when you are smiling. Even if you don't feel like smiling, do it anyway. Smiling will make you feel better and give you more reason to smile again. It may feel stupid at first, but try it. It really works.

PLAY MUSIC. Research has shown that music can have strong effects on our moods. Our favorite music will put us in a good mood. When you are feeling down or overwhelmed, or when it seems your baby just won't stop crying, listen to some favorite music. Put on soft, soothing music if you are feeling stressed. Put on fun, energetic music if you don't feel that you have the energy to go on. It is a great way to motivate yourself to clean the house or just to dance. It will help put older children in a good mood too. Get everyone into the dancing mode.

A CALM PARENT EQUALS A CALM BABY

Your baby will sense your mood. If you are upset, she will be upset. If you are tense, she will be tense. But if you are happy, she will be happy.

Your baby looks to you for cues on how to react to the world. If you start to feel tense as bedtime is approaching, your baby is going to sense that and think there is something she should be worried about and afraid of. However, if you approach bedtime with a feeling of serenity, she will sense this and feel serene as well.

RELAXATION STRATEGIES

Psychologists have had a great deal of success in developing techniques that help people relax in stressful situations. People with anxiety disorders, people about to undergo a stressful medical procedure, or those who need to learn stress-management techniques often use these strategies. Try out a few and decide what works best for you to help you cope when dealing with an upset baby.

Progressive Muscle Relaxation

Some say that progressive muscle relaxation (PMR) is the gold standard of relaxation strategies. It takes practice, but once learned it is an excellent way to reduce stress. Progressive muscle relaxation teaches you to identify and relieve tension in your muscles. When you are stressed or upset, you may not even notice how much you are tensing your muscles. This technique will help you identify times when you are tense and teach you to relax.

In PMR, each muscle is sequentially tensed and relaxed to help you identify tension and then release it. In the beginning, progressive muscle relaxation takes between twenty and thirty minutes. The more you practice, the less time it will take. By the end you will be able to relax in a matter of moments.

Follow the script outlined below. You can tape it on a tape recorder if you want. However, if you are like many people who don't like to hear the sound of their own voices, get someone else to do this for you. The person should speak in a slow, soothing manner. The exact words used are not important; it is the process that is important. You don't even need to follow a script as long as you sequentially tense and relax your muscles. Each time that you tense a muscle, keep it tensed for about ten seconds.

How do you feel after progressive muscle relaxation? You should feel extremely relaxed. Continue to practice. That is the only way to get good at this technique. Even if you feel completely relaxed after the first time, you will feel more and more relaxed each time you practice. After a number of sessions (over at least two weeks),

Progressive Muscle Relaxation Script

MUSCLE GROUP	TENSING EXERCISE
Lower arms	Make a fist
Upper arms	Make a muscle
Lower legs	Point toes
Thighs	Squeeze legs together
Stomach	Tighten stomach muscles
Chest	Take a deep breath
Shoulders	Raise shoulders to ears
Neck	Lower chin to chest
Jaw	Bite down firmly
Lips	Press lips together
Eyes	Close eyes tightly
Forehead	Frown, draw eyebrows together

To begin this exercise, find a comfortable position, perhaps lying on a bed or sitting in a reclining chair. Remove your glasses (if you wear them), get comfortable, and close your eyes. Keep your eyes closed throughout the relaxation process.

Here is a sample script that you can use to practice progressive muscle relaxation.

Begin by taking a few deep breaths. Breathe relaxation in and breathe tension out.
(Wait 20 seconds.)

Now tense the muscles of your right hand by making a fist. Feel the tension . . . study the tension . . . and relax. Notice the difference between the tension and the relaxation.
(Wait 20 seconds.)

Now tense the muscles of your right arm by making a muscle. Feel the tension . . . study the tension . . . and relax. Notice the difference.
(Wait 5 seconds.)

Just let yourself become more and more relaxed. Feel your muscles becoming loose . . . heavy . . . and relaxed. Just let your muscles go.
(Wait 5 seconds.)

Now tense the muscles of your left hand by making a fist. Feel the tension . . . study the tension . . . and relax. Notice the difference between the tension and the relaxation.
(Wait 20 seconds.)

Now tense the muscles of your left arm by making a muscle. Feel the tension . . . study the tension . . . and relax. Notice the difference.
(Wait 5 seconds.)

You are becoming more and more relaxed, sleepy and relaxed.
(Wait 5 seconds.)

Now tense the muscles of your right leg by pointing your toes. Feel the tension . . . study the tension . . . and relax. Notice the difference between the tension and the relaxation.
(Wait 20 seconds.)

Now tense the muscles of your left leg by pointing your toes. Feel the tension . . . study the tension . . . and relax. Notice the difference.
(Wait 5 seconds.)

Just continue to relax.
(Wait 5 seconds.)

Now tense the muscles of your upper legs by pressing your thighs together. Feel the tension . . . study the tension . . . and relax. Notice the difference between the tension and the relaxation.
(Wait 20 seconds.)

Now tense the muscles of your stomach. Feel the tension . . . study the tension . . . and relax. Notice the difference.
(Wait 5 seconds.)

The relaxation is becoming deeper and deeper. You are feeling relaxed, drowsy and relaxed. With each breath in, your relaxation increases. With each exhalation, you spread the relaxation throughout your body.
(Wait 5 seconds.)

Now tense the muscles of your chest by taking a deep breath. Feel the tension . . . study the tension . . . and exhale. Notice the difference between the tension and the relaxation.
(Wait 20 seconds.)

Now tense the muscles of your shoulders by hunching your shoulders toward your ears. Feel the tension . . . study the tension . . . and relax. Notice the difference.
(Wait 5 seconds.)

Let yourself become more and more relaxed.
(Wait 5 seconds.)

Now tense the muscles of your jaw by biting down firmly. Feel the tension . . . study the tension . . . and relax. Notice the difference between the tension and the relaxation.
(Wait 20 seconds.)

Now tense the muscles of your lower face by pressing your lips together firmly. Feel the tension . . . study the tension . . . and relax. Notice the difference.
(Wait 5 seconds.)

Now the very deep state of relaxation is moving through all the areas of your body as your muscles completely relax.
(Wait 5 seconds.)

Now tense the muscles of your eyes by closing them tightly. Feel the tension . . . study the tension . . . and exhale. Notice the difference between the tension and the relaxation.
(Wait 20 seconds.)

Now tense the muscles of your forehead by frowning and drawing your eyebrows together. Feel the tension . . . study the tension . . . and relax. Notice the difference.
(Wait 5 seconds.)

Let yourself become more and more relaxed.
(Wait 20 seconds.)

Now relax all the muscles of your body; just let them become more and more relaxed.
(Wait 20 seconds.)

Remain in your very relaxed state. Begin to notice your breathing. Breathe through your nose. Notice the cool air as you breathe in and the warm moist air as you exhale. Just continue to notice your breathing. Now each time you exhale, mentally repeat the word "relax." Inhale, exhale, relax . . . inhale, exhale, relax.
(Wait 20 seconds.)

Now you are going to return to your normal, alert state. As I count backward, you will gradually become more alert. When I reach "two," open your eyes. When I get to "one," you will be entirely alert. Five . . . four . . . you are becoming more alert . . . three . . . you feel very refreshed . . . two . . . now open your eyes . . . one.

cut back the number of muscle groups by half (tense and relax both fists together, both arms together, both legs together, then the thighs, chest, neck, lips, eyes). Practice again for two weeks. Cut back the muscle groups again by half (both arms, both legs, chest, lips). By now you should be an expert at becoming relaxed. Once you are good at PMR, the word "relax" will be well associated with a completely relaxed state. Use the word "relax" in your everyday life to help you relax in tense situations. It is a good time to try it when the baby is crying.

Diaphragmatic Breathing

Slow, even breathing is also an excellent way to relax. Many people breathe shallowly from their upper chest. This type of breathing can cause you to hyperventilate. A better way to breathe is from your diaphragm. This technique will take only a few moments to learn.

First, lie down on your back on the floor or on a firm bed. Place your hand on your chest and breathe using your chest muscles so that you feel your chest rise and fall with each breath. Keeping that hand on your chest, place your other hand on your stomach. Continue to breathe from your chest and feel that your stomach muscles hardly move. Now breathe from your diaphragm. This will require you to take deeper breaths. When you breathe from your diaphragm, your chest will hardly move and your stomach will rise and fall. Continue doing this for a few minutes and get the feel of it. Once you think you have it, sit up, leaving your hands in place on your chest and stomach. Continue to practice diaphragmatic breathing, that is, breathing from your diaphragm. When you are ready, stand up and continue to breathe from your diaphragm. Again, keep your hands where they are while you get the hang of it. If you think that you lost the feeling for the process, return to a lying position.

In the beginning, when you go to use this technique, you will need to place your hand on your stomach to make sure that you are breathing from your diaphragm. As you get better at it, you will no longer need to do this. When doing diaphragmatic breathing, take slow, deep breaths. Don't breathe too fast, or you may hyperventilate, which will make you feel even more stressed. Take several deep breaths. Then breathe normally. Take several deep breaths again. Within a few minutes you should feel calmer and more ready to face the world—or at least a crying baby.

Diaphragmatic breathing is an excellent stress reducer in any situation. If you are about to give a presentation at work and are feeling stressed, do your diaphragmatic breathing. Upset with your spouse and feeling stressed? Do a few minutes of deep breathing. This type of deep breathing can be done anywhere. No one will even know that you are performing a stress relaxation technique. You can do it at home, while in a store, or out at a restaurant. Deep breathing will send messages to your body to calm down. It will change your body's reaction to stress.

Guided Imagery

Guided imagery is another excellent way to relax. At times, we all imagine ourselves to be somewhere else. If you imagine yourself in a stressful situation, such as having to make a stressful presentation or being in danger, you will become tense. Your body will react as if you were actually in that situation. Your heart will pound, your pulse will race, and you may feel jittery all over. This will also happen if you imagine yourself listening to your baby crying. If you imagine yourself in a pleasant, relaxing scene, your breathing will become more even and your pulse will slow. Imagining yourself in such a pleasant situation will therefore help you to relax.

The first thing you will need to do is develop a pleasant scenario. Lie back, close your eyes, and think of your favorite place. For example, this is the scene that Michael developed for himself: "I am lying on the beach in Hawaii. The sun is warm. The beach is quiet. I can hear a few people talking and laughing in the distance. I can hear the waves crashing. I can smell the salt water in the air and hear the birds. The sand is warm under my hands, and my whole body is relaxed, relishing the moment." Michael is able to think of this scene any time that he is feeling stressed. He thinks of it when he begins worrying about finances or is in a stressful meeting at work. He can even go there in his mind when his baby has been screaming for twenty minutes.

Maybe your relaxing place is on top of a mountain or sitting in front of a fireplace. Whatever your scene, think of it using all your senses. What do you hear? What do you smell? What do you feel? The more senses that you engage, the easier it will be to imagine. Once you have developed your scene, imagine yourself there two to three times a day. Embellish it until you can actually feel yourself there. With practice you will be able to imagine yourself in your peaceful setting almost instantaneously and will quickly feel relaxed. When the baby is crying or you are stuck in traffic, put yourself at your scene and enjoy the sensation.

Other Relaxation Strategies

There are many other ways that people relax. Some people do yoga. Others meditate. Whatever works for you, do it. Being relaxed is important for your mental well-being. It will help you cope with teaching your baby to sleep on his own, and amazingly, it will make the process go faster and more smoothly. The calmer you are, the calmer your baby will be, and a calm baby will quickly become a sleeping baby.

CHALLENGE THOSE THOUGHTS

Our thoughts are very powerful. What we are thinking can make us feel happy or can make us feel stressed. Dealing with a crying baby, especially one who won't sleep, makes us think negative thoughts. Imagine that it has been forty minutes of constant crying for the second night in a row. You might start thinking, "This is never going to work." Everyone thinks that at some point. Your thoughts may be irrational: "He is never going to stop crying" or "It's not fair that my baby won't sleep when everyone else's does." You may be angry with your baby for not sleeping and not letting you sleep. Such thoughts make it even harder to cope with the situation. Do you get caught up in negative thoughts that are just making you feel worse? Your negative thoughts are not going to make the baby stop crying or start sleeping. Instead, they are going to make the situation worse. Your baby will sense your stress and become even more upset. To get out of the vicious cycle of your thoughts affecting how you feel, you need to combat your negative beliefs.

The first step to combating negative thoughts is to notice what you are thinking. Write your thoughts down. You may be surprised at the ideas that are going through your head. Once you have identified your thoughts, you can begin to challenge them. Argue with yourself. Present the logical side: "My baby will stop crying. Eventually he will have to fall asleep" or "I am not a failure as a parent simply because my baby has problems sleeping. Otherwise, my baby is happy and healthy" or "My baby's not sleeping is not my fault, and it is not his fault. He has simply gotten into some bad habits" or "Why would this program not work for my baby? It has worked for so many other babies. I can do it."

Teaching your baby to sleep through the night is not an easy process. It takes work and will probably involve some tears (likely on everyone's part). When you notice that you are thinking negative thoughts, combat them. Stress the positive: "This is going to work" or "It is only the second night. Next week at this time everyone will be sleeping." By saying positive things you will feel better and will be better able to cope.

GET SLEEP YOURSELF

One important issue for both you and your partner is to make sure that you get some sleep. It is very difficult to cope with anything when you are sleep deprived. Try to work out a system with your partner to share the child care duties so each of you can get as much sleep as possible.

For example, one person can take late-night duty, and the other can be "on" in the morning. That way one person can get to sleep early at night, and the other can sleep in the next morning. This solution worked well in our family with our daughter. Since I was nursing, I would pump at 9:00 at night and then head to bed. My husband would then do a scheduled feeding with a bottle of pumped breast milk around 11:00 p.m. Thus, he took over the first part of the night, so I was able to get about five hours of sleep before taking over at the next feeding, around 2:30 a.m. After that point, I would get up to take care of the baby when necessary. That way each of us got at least five uninterrupted hours of sleep, plus several more disrupted hours. Of course, it helped that my husband is a night owl and I am an early bird. If that is the situation in your family, take advantage of it.

Another option is to swap off nights: take turns getting up with the baby. On weekends, one parent can do Friday night and the other Saturday night. Be forewarned, though, that two problems can occur when using this system. The first is that the parent who is on duty does not wake up when the baby cries. By the time the partner who is on duty wakes up (or is awakened), the other partner may already be wide awake and may as well take care of the baby. If that happens, wake your on-duty partner and make him or her get up. Put the baby monitor on that person's side of the bed. If you continue to get up and take care of the baby, your partner will learn to sleep through the noise and will never wake to the cries, so it is important that the on-duty person be awakened. With a little training the adult on duty should begin to wake when the baby does.

The other issue is what to do when one parent works and the other parent stays home. Usually in this type of situation, the person who remains at home always gets up with the baby because the other person is expected to function at work the next day. But people do not always realize how much work it is to stay home with a baby. Taking care of a baby or a toddler takes enormous effort, physically and emotionally. A fairer solution is to compromise, but the compromise does not have to be exactly fifty-fifty. The working partner (in the more traditional sense) can take over on Thursday nights, when only one day is left in the workweek, and on weekends. Another solution is for the working person to take every third night rather than every other night. At the very least, the working parent can take the duty on the weekends to give the stay-at-home partner a break. Working out a solution for this problem is important. We all need sufficient sleep to be at our best. The working parent also benefits from solving this problem because he or she will not be coming home to an overtired and cranky partner.

If you are a single parent, getting sleep yourself is going to be even more of a challenge. Try to get some extra sleep during the day; nap when your baby naps. It can be very helpful to get some assistance at night. Have a friend or a relative sleep over a night or two a week to give you a break. It may be beneficial to hire a babysitter who comes at night, either in addition to help during the day or instead of daytime hours.

COPING WITH LOSS OF SLEEP

If you are sleepy, be careful. Don't take long drives in the car (some moms and dads even fall asleep on short drives!). Be careful in the kitchen and when doing other chores, such as yard work. Accidents can happen when you are tired. Often we are expected to get things done no matter how much sleep we got the night before, the week before, or even the month before. Before you just jump in and do whatever is expected, think about whether or not you realistically can. Will you be safe? Will you be endangering others? For example, more car accidents are caused by driving when sleepy than by driving while intoxicated. These accidents are more likely to occur in the middle of the night, as you might expect. But, surprisingly, the next most dangerous time is between three and five in the afternoon. Turning up the radio or rolling down the car window to get a blast of fresh air is not going to help much in preventing you from falling asleep at the wheel. The only thing to do is stop and take a quick nap, even if just for ten to fifteen minutes. Of course, if you can take a longer nap, do so. If you are not getting enough sleep, figure out the limits of what you can reasonably and safely achieve.

Reminders

+ Teaching a baby to sleep through the night can be stressful for parents.
+ There are many ways to cope, including using humor, adjusting your thinking, and remaining calm.
+ Relaxation strategies, including progressive muscle relaxation, diaphragmatic breathing, and guided imagery, are all excellent ways to deal with stressful situations.
+ Strategize ways to get sleep yourself.

CHAPTER 10

"What Do I Do If...?": Dealing with Difficult Situations

"I tried to get Peter to sleep through the night, but breast-feeding makes everything more difficult."

"I tried sleep training, but when Gregory climbed out of the crib, I gave up."

Some parents fail to change their child's sleep habits because of a particular situation, such as breast-feeding, or because something unexpected occurs, such as their child climbing out of the crib or vomiting. Many of the parents I see in my clinical practice do not know what to do when something unexpected occurs. I find it is helpful to have parents develop a plan for solving every situation that they think could possibly occur.

"HE HATES HIS CRIB"

Julia is sure that her nineteen-month-old son, Lucas, hates his crib. Every night he wakes up at 2:00 a.m. and screams until one of his parents comes in to get him and brings him to their bed.

Sondra is sure Nakeem hates his crib. She tries putting him down in his crib once he is fast asleep. Inevitably, he wakes up and starts crying. Eventually, she gives up and sits in a rocking chair holding him for most of the night.

You can't imagine how often I hear parents proclaim that their child hates his or her crib. This statement is often followed by the question of whether all of their child's sleep problems will be resolved if they simply switch their child to a bed. The answer is almost always "No!" Rather, such a switch usually makes sleep problems worse. Children rarely hate their cribs. They don't have any context for hating their cribs. They may hate getting their diaper changed because they have to lie still, or they may hate zucchini because it tastes yucky, but they do not typically hate their cribs. What they actually are having a problem with is going to sleep on their own, rather than being rocked to sleep, held to sleep, or whatever has been their lifelong habit of falling asleep. Thus, a move to a bed has no impact on this change, and the freedom to roam often makes things worse.

Luciene found this to be true when she moved her fourteen-month-old daughter to a toddler bed. Sasha had always fallen asleep on the living room couch and cried when she was put in her crib. When Luciene got a toddler bed, Sasha protested being in the bed, too, and would come stomping out of the bedroom every time her mother tried to leave. It wasn't the crib that Sasha was protesting; it was falling asleep in her room rather than on the living room couch while watching television.

Rather than make a drastic change from a crib to a bed, work on establishing good sleep habits and having your child soothe herself to sleep at bedtime (see Chapter 6 for lots more information on this topic). As a first step to get your child accustomed to her crib (and to her room), spend time throughout the day playing in and around her crib. Take five to ten minutes several times a day and play games involving the crib. Hide her favorite teddy bear in her crib and find it together. At first hold her while you "discover" the toy in her crib. Then hold her while she finds the teddy. Very quickly you'll be able to move to putting your little one into the crib to get the teddy bear herself. Play peekaboo, with you looking through the rails of the crib at her. You will quickly notice a major difference in your child's attitude toward the crib. She'll discover that it is a fun place. At the same time that you are doing fun daytime activities that involve the crib, start doing your child's bedtime routine in her room, taking her where she normally falls asleep as the last step (such as in your bed or in your arms). Both of these steps will set the foundation for her falling asleep on her own in her crib.

CLIMBING OUT OF THE CRIB

Billy is two years old. He has just figured out how to get out of his crib. He puts his right foot up on the rail and pulls himself over. The first two times that he did this he fell down and banged his head on the floor. He has since become an expert and can climb out swiftly and easily. It has gotten to the point where he climbs out the moment he is put down for a nap or at bedtime.

Maggie is three years old. She had never even tried to climb out of her crib. The other day, though, Maggie suddenly appeared at the top of the stairs at the end of her nap, yelling, "I'm done!"

There are two groups of toddlers: those who climb out of their crib and those who don't. Some babies try to climb out of their crib as early as eighteen months of age. Other children won't even attempt it until they are at least two and a half. And then there are those who never do. Ideally, your toddler will never try this stunt. Climbing out of the crib is something that understandably causes many parents concern. They worry that their child may get hurt, and because they don't know what to do when it happens.

A parent's immediate reaction often is to give up on using a crib and move the toddler to a bed. This doesn't have to be the answer. There are other solutions to this problem. But first, make sure that your child will not get harmed if he does decide to take the leap. Put pillows on the floor around the crib. Remove any nearby objects, such as toys or pieces of furniture (especially toy chests), on which your child can bang his head.

Here are some suggestions that many parents have found helpful.

LOWER THE MATTRESS. Move the crib mattress to its lowest setting to make climbing impossible. If your child can't physically manage to climb out, he won't. This works especially well for younger toddlers or when your child is small in size.

REMOVE ALL CRIB TOYS AND BUMPERS. Take all large toys out of the crib, as well as the crib bumpers if they are still in the crib, so your toddler can't use these as a step stool to give him a boost up and over.

DON'T MAKE IT WORTH IT. The major reason babies climb out of their cribs is that they get something out of it. Don't let your child climb in bed with you after climbing out.

DON'T GIVE HIM LOTS OF ATTENTION. Very calmly and neutrally return your child to his crib and say in a firm voice, "No climbing." After several more attempts, your child will realize that climbing out is not worth it. He is just going to be put right back in his crib.

BE FIRM. This is not a behavior about which you can be wishy-washy. There is too high a risk that your toddler will hurt himself. Don't let him rule the roost just because he climbed out once. Take a stance, set limits, and be firm.

CATCH 'EM EARLY. If your child makes a habit of climbing out of the crib, catch him at it early. Stand where you can see him, but he can't see you. The moment your child starts to put his foot on the rail or over the rail, say immediately and firmly, "No climbing." If you startle your child enough and do it several times, he will stop trying to climb out.

INSTALL A CRIB TENT. Many manufacturers make mesh crib tents. (See Appendix B, "Resources for Parents," for places to purchase these tents.) These tents attach to the crib rails with Velcro. They work great to deter little climbers, making it impossible for them to climb out. They are simple to install, and it is still easy to get to your child quickly. Parents swear by them, as they keep little ones snug and safe. The tents can also be used to keep pets out of your baby's crib.

WHEN ALL ELSE FAILS. If you have exhausted all other remedies, you may want to lower the side bar and push a stool up next to the crib to prevent a bad fall. This way your child has a safe way to get out of the crib and doesn't have such a great distance to cover to get to the floor. If your child is likely to start wandering around the house, install a gate at the bedroom door. You can also attach a bell to the bedroom door to alert you that your child is trying to leave his bedroom. This may be even more important if your bedroom is on a different floor from your child's room.

GETTING OUT OF BED

It is much more difficult to teach your child to be a good sleeper when he is in a bed rather than in a crib. He is now more mobile. He can get out of bed whenever he wants. This may occur once, twice, or seventeen times in one evening.

Thinking back to Chapter 6, remember that the trick to having your child sleep through the night and fall asleep easily at bedtime is to teach him to fall asleep on his own *in his own bed.* Amazingly, most children do stay in their bed when they make the move from a crib (see Chapter 11 for more information on switching from a crib to a bed). Your child, however, may be one of those who simply will not stay put.

As discussed in Chapter 3, the two basic principles of changing your child's behavior are to use reinforcement and be consistent. Oh, yes, and remain calm—which is probably the hardest part. Decide on a night when you are going to start insisting that your child remain in his bed. Do it on a night that you don't have to get other things done, such as pay bills or make phone calls, because this may take a while. You may even want to start when you know you have several nights to devote to this endeavor.

First, perform your bedtime routine. Put your child to bed and leave the room. When he gets out of bed, calmly return him to bed and tell him that he must stay in bed. When he is in bed, tell him what a good boy he is for being in bed. Say good night and leave the room. Do this again and again and again. Remain calm. Keep your interaction with your child to a minimum. You want to reinforce him for being in bed, not for getting out of bed. If he is getting something from his behavior, such as more attention or upsetting you, he is more likely to do it again. After numerous times if you stay calm, consistent, and firm, he'll get the message: Getting out of bed is simply not worth it. On those occasions when he has remained in bed after you left, go back in and praise him for staying in bed.

On night two, repeat the process. Don't be surprised if it takes longer on the second night. To your child, the first night may have been a fluke, and he will want to let you know that he is not kidding. He does not want to stay in bed. He will test the limits. Be strong and stick to your plan. If you eventually give in and allow him to stay out of bed, you are going to have quite a battle on your hands in the future. You will have taught your child that if he is persistent, you will eventually give in, and he will then keep getting out of bed.

Some parents have found that staying close to their child's room will help their child stay in bed. He will know that you are close by. If you choose this method, stay shorter and shorter periods of time. Start by staying for fifteen minutes. Decrease the amount of time that you stay by two or three minutes per night. Within a week you can probably leave easily. For more anxious children, this process may take several weeks. This method can be extremely useful if you have recently moved to a new house or if your child is sleeping in a strange place.

COMING OUT OF THE BEDROOM

Your child may not only leave his bed, but also his room. When this happens, follow the same routine as when he gets out of bed. There are also other ways to keep your child in his bedroom. One method that has been successful for many families is to install a bell or an alarm that rings when their child tries to come out of his room. Bells that hang over doorways or burglar alarms that go off when the doorknob is touched are inexpensive and easy to install. This way you will know that your child is out of his room. This can be very helpful for a family where the child wakes in the middle of the night and leaves his bedroom without the parents being aware of it. Many parents comment that they wake up in the morning only to find their child in bed with them. If this doesn't bother you, then fine. If it does, you will need to devise some system to awaken you when your child is up and wandering.

A baby gate in your child's doorway will help keep your child in his room and can be especially useful with toddlers. If you do put up a gate, explain to your child that when the gate is up, it is a reminder that it is nighttime (or naptime), and when the gate is down, that lets him know that it is time to get up.

Parents often wonder whether they should lock the door to their child's room. For some families, locking the door is easier than holding the door shut and getting into a power play with their child. An alternative to locking the door is to tell your child that if he is in bed, the door stays unlocked or even partially open. Once he gets out of bed, however, the door gets locked. If you are going to do this, be consistent. The moment your child is back in bed unlock or open the door.

Locking the door has many drawbacks, however. First, it can be dangerous. If there is a fire or an emergency, your child cannot get out. If you lock the door only to keep your child in his room at bedtime, unlock it once you know that he is asleep. Another problem is that your child can get hurt when left in a room without supervision. Make sure that there is nothing in the bedroom that can injure your child. Remove all dangerous objects. Your child may also destroy the room. You may return to the room to find your child asleep on the floor and everything pulled out of the closet and every drawer overturned. Last, and most important, locking the door can be very scary to a child. Before you resort to locking the door, try alternative methods, and be firm and consistent.

GETTING UNDRESSED

Laura is two and a half. She has always been a good sleeper, going to bed without a problem at 7:30 and sleeping until 7:00 in the morning. When she wakes in the morning, she plays in her crib quietly and happily for another half hour. She naps every afternoon for two hours. Laura's mother, Alicia, considers herself lucky. In the past few weeks, however, Laura has begun stripping off all her clothes and her diaper in her crib. She has done this several times in the morning and during many of her naps. Unfortunately, she is also not toilet trained, which means the crib is often soaked. Amazingly, whenever Alicia goes in to get Laura, Laura immediately begins telling her mother, "C-c-cold," and doing a shivering routine. But this hasn't stopped Laura from getting undressed.

Young children usually undress either because they are bored or to get attention. If your child is wide-awake when put to bed or wakes earlier than everyone else in the morning, she may undress to keep herself amused. This may mean that you are leaving her in the crib too long in the morning or at naptime, or you are putting her to bed too early, before she is tired at night.

If your baby is getting undressed because she is bored, put lots of toys in her crib to keep her amused. If she throws her toys out of the crib, attach a busy box to the crib rails or hang interesting objects from a mobile. You can even change these objects frequently to hold her interest. If your child is under the age of one year, be sure and remove the toys once she is asleep to avoid SIDS.

If she gets undressed to get your attention, ignore the behavior. In a few days, when getting undressed doesn't get your attention, she will stop. At that point it won't be worth it to her anymore.

Another way to deal with your child's getting undressed is similar to the advice given above for climbing out of the crib. Stand where your child can't see you. The moment that she begins to undress herself say "no" in a firm, loud voice. As long as you are consistent, the undressing should stop.

Some parents have resorted to putting their child in clothes that she can't unfasten. Also, some pajamas can be turned around so that all fasteners are in the back, where little hands can't reach. (Obviously, you won't be able to turn feet pajamas around.)

PACIFIERS

If your child uses a pacifier to self-soothe, she may get into trouble when the pacifier gets lost. This problem usually occurs in the first six months. After six or seven months, most babies have the physical capability to find their pacifiers and get it into their mouths. If your baby is younger than six months, you have two choices. One choice is to wait it out, going in and getting your baby her pacifier until she is able to retrieve it herself. The other choice is to take the pacifier away altogether and have your child learn to sleep without it. When making this choice, you may want to start with a week of just taking it away at bedtime and continuing to give it to your baby at naptime and during the night. This will help everyone get some sleep. In a week, it's no more pacifier.

The first approach—hanging in there until your baby is six or seven months old—is recommended. Some babies have a high need to suck, and pacifiers meet that need. Also, once a baby is able to find her pacifier, she usually becomes a great sleeper, especially if you restrict pacifier use to sleep times only. You'll find your toddler diving for her crib to get to her pacifier. In the morning and at the end of naptime, make a game of tossing down the pacifier before getting out of the crib.

Once your baby is six or seven months old, she will likely have the dexterity to find her pacifier and get it herself. Strategically place a bunch of pacifiers in one corner of her crib. If one gets lost or thrown out of the crib, she should be able to find another one without your assistance. When you put your baby in her crib at bedtime, have her reach for the pacifier on her own. During the night, also encourage her to get her pacifier. For the first week or so, you may have to put your hand on hers and guide her. After a week or two, simply encourage her: "Get your binky [or whatever you call it]." You can also spend playtime during the day practicing getting the pacifier. Put your baby on the floor and play "pacifier pickup," putting the pacifier next to your baby and encouraging her to find it.

Do not tie pacifiers to the slats of the crib, because this can be dangerous. Babies can strangle themselves on the string, especially if they roll over with the pacifier in their mouth.

GETTING RID OF THE PACIFIER. There are many conflicting opinions on when it's time to get rid of the pacifier. Many pediatricians and pediatric dentists have differing opinions. Some believe that you should do it by fifteen months, whereas others say two years, and still others four years. My recommendation is four years.

Before that time, your child is likely to have a hard time adjusting to sleeping without the pacifier, and the transition to give it up may be much harder on him. Take it away too early and you could have weeks of sobbing for the binky. Also, if you take it away too early, your child may switch to sucking his thumb, which is a much more difficult habit to break later on. Don't take away the pacifier when you are about to go through other major developmental changes, such as toilet training, moving from a crib to a big bed, or starting preschool. At four, your child will be cognitively ready to give up the pacifier, although he may still miss it. Have the "binky fairy" come during the night and take away the pacifiers, leaving a present behind. Don't wait too much longer after four years, as then pacifier use can interfere with the placement of permanent teeth. Once the pacifier is gone, you may be surprised at how much your child's baby teeth will move back into place.

BREAST-FEEDING

Seven-month-old Peter falls asleep each night between 7:00 and 8:00 while nursing. Tara, his mother, usually goes to bed shortly after Peter because she knows that he generally wakes at about 11:30 and again between 2:00 and 3:00 in the morning. Each time she nurses him back to sleep.

As mentioned in Chapter 2, there are several reasons why breast-fed babies take longer to sleep through the night than bottle-fed babies. Since breast milk is easier to digest than formula, a breast-fed baby will digest the milk faster and get hungry again quicker, resulting in a shorter time span between feedings. You may therefore find yourself needing to wake more times during the night to breast-feed your baby. Keep in mind, though, that once your baby is six months old (for some babies, it's much earlier), he is getting enough nutrition during the day and doesn't need to breast-feed during the night. Check with your pediatrician if you are concerned about your child's growth or wonder whether your child still needs middle-of-the-night feedings.

In addition, breast-fed babies often have a strong association between nursing and falling asleep. As a longtime nursing mother myself, I understand how easily this happens. Nursing is a wonderful sedative, both for baby and for Mom. It can get you into trouble, though, when your baby can't fall asleep without it.

The key to solving the problem is to eliminate the association between feeding and falling asleep. Here are several strategies.

DECREASE BREAST-FEEDING GRADUALLY. As discussed in Chapter 6, one solution that has worked for many nursing mothers is to decrease the length of time that they breast-feed at naptimes and bedtime. To do this, you will need to time how long you usually breast-feed at bedtime. If you usually nurse for ten minutes, decrease breast-feeding by one minute each subsequent night: on night one, nurse for nine minutes; on night two, eight minutes; and so forth. End at either two or three minutes of nursing. (It is too much of a tease to nurse for just one minute.) If you usually nurse for a very long time at bedtime, you may want to decrease by two minutes each night.

CHANGE THE TIME YOU NURSE. Rather than wean your child gradually, simply change the time that you breast-feed so it is not near the time that your child usually falls asleep. Nurse when your baby awakens from a nap rather than when he falls asleep. Nurse first thing in the morning. If you usually breast-feed your baby at 7:30, expecting him to be asleep and in his crib between 7:45 and 8:00, breast-feed instead at 6:30 and have an hour of quiet playtime before getting ready for bed. Or simply move nursing earlier in your bedtime routine. Nurse first, and then do bath and books.

INVOLVE OTHERS. Get someone else involved in putting your baby to sleep and responding to him in the middle of the night. You can ask the baby's father, a sitter, a friend, or a grandparent to rock your baby to sleep and go to him during the night when he wakes. Once your baby no longer needs to nurse to sleep, you can get involved again in the bedtime routine. Your baby will have developed other soothing techniques and have other ways to cope with going back to sleep besides just wanting to nurse.

WAKE THE BABY. I know, I can hear you saying: "Wake a sleeping baby? Are you crazy?" Yes, wake the baby. If your baby falls asleep while you are nursing him, wake him before putting him in his crib. Change his diaper, burp him, or read a story. Put him in his crib awake so that he puts himself to sleep. Your baby may not like having you wake him and may even cry, but this will last for only a short time. In a few days you will not need to breast-feed at sleep times and can simply put him in his crib awake.

"JUST ONE MORE"

"Just one more hug."
"One more story."
"I need a drink of water."

Children ask for "one more" for several reasons. They may actually want a drink of water, or they may have forgotten to bring to bed their favorite stuffed animal. They may do it to make sure that you really are nearby when you promised you would be and will come if they need help. They may do it to avoid going to sleep, especially if they think that you are having fun without them. And, of course, they may do it for attention. Even if you scold them, that is still attention—not as much fun as positive attention, but attention nonetheless.

How should you deal with this? First, try to figure out exactly why your child is doing this. If she really just needs her covers straightened, she will do it rarely and will stop calling you once the problem is solved. If your child seems nervous that you are not around or because she can't see you, she may really need to know that you are nearby. For these children, simply responding to them verbally by saying something like, "It's okay. Go to sleep" may do the trick. Some children may not actually be sleepy enough to go to bed, so try moving bedtime later by thirty minutes or so. For those children who simply don't want to go to bed or are getting rewarded for their bedtime behavior, you will have to set some limits.

First of all, children should always get one chance. Even if your child always calls for "one more" at bedtime, she may actually really need to go to the bathroom or need her favorite doll. Responding to her once will let her know that you really are there when she needs you. After that, be firm. Reply that now it is time to go to sleep. Be neutral. Don't yell. Don't lose your temper. Remember, yelling is still attention even if doesn't seem fun to you. (Make sure you read Chapter 3 on how to manage children's behavior.) Some families have found using a "bedtime card" to be helpful. Your child can turn in the card for a request, such as a drink of water or going and saying good night to the cat. Once the card has been turned in, no more requests are allowed.

If you say, "This is the last time," mean it. Those words carry no weight if you are willing to return when your child calls or will come in and pick up the dropped pacifier numerous times. Rebecca, twenty-two months, knew that dropping her pacifier out of her crib always got her parents' attention. Her parents owned a video baby monitor, so Rebecca would look directly at the camera, smile, and drop her pacifier overboard.

You also have to remember that children love rules, and they love to have limits set. After testing the rules and understanding how far they can go, they will understand what they are supposed to do and be better behaved.

VOMITING

Anne is the mother of fifteen-month-old Harry, who has rarely, if ever, slept through the night. On the first night implementing the changes suggested in Chapter 6, everything went smoothly and according to plan. On night two, however, Harry cried so hard that he vomited all over himself and his crib. Anne ran into Harry's room, took him out of his crib, cleaned him up, and rocked him to sleep. After that, Anne was afraid to leave him for too long or to allow him to cry for more than five minutes because she was concerned that he would vomit again.

Some children vomit after crying for a long period, and it is understandably very upsetting to parents. Unfortunately, however, some young children learn to vomit at will if the vomiting is reinforced by attention. Some young children get to the point where they chronically vomit every time they are upset or do not get their way, as it gets parents to respond. This can be a real problem.

Vomiting can be dealt with just like any other behavior. If your baby vomits after crying, don't worry too much about it and don't reinforce it. Be neutral. Change the sheets, clean up the baby as well as you can (preferably without picking him up), and leave the room. One helpful hint is to make up your baby's crib with two sets of sheets (with a liner in between) so that if he vomits, you can quickly and easily take off the top set and leave the bottom set on. Sheets that fasten to the bars of the crib with Velcro and all-in-one sheets also make this process easier (see Appendix B, "Resources for Parents," for places that sell these sheets).

If, however, your child is vomiting at other times of the day, you should call your pediatrician. If bedtime is the only time he vomits and he has appeared fine all day, it is likely to be a behavioral problem rather than a medical problem.

CRIES EVERY TIME

Even after three weeks of sleep training, Alexis still cries every night at bedtime. She'll usually cry for about five minutes, but sometimes cries for as long as fifteen minutes. Elena finds it very upsetting.

Most babies start falling asleep quickly without fussing within a week. Others may take two weeks. But there are some babies who are still upset at bedtime after two weeks. There are many reasons why babies continue to fuss at bedtime.

+ **Takes longer.** For some babies, sleep training just takes a bit longer. These are usually babies whose parents describe them as "willful." All changes seem to take a while and are met with some resistance. For these babies, being consistent and giving it a bit more time will resolve the problem.
+ **Overtired.** Other babies continue to cry at bedtime because they are overtired and are having a hard time settling down. Moving bedtime earlier can make a huge improvement.
+ **Inconsistency.** If you are being inconsistent in how you respond to your child, sometimes going in and getting your baby and other times leaving her, she'll likely continue to cry at bedtime to see what happens. Be more consistent. Check on her, but be clear that it is time to go night-night.
+ **Last gasp.** There are some babies who will always fuss at bedtime. It seems to be a final letting go of steam before

conking out. Basically, it's the last gasp before crashing for the night.

MY CHILD STILL WAKES UP AT NIGHT

As stated previously, most infants and toddlers will naturally start sleeping through the night within two weeks or so of falling asleep easily and quickly at bedtime, but not all! So, what should you do if your baby still doesn't sleep through the night even after several weeks of her going to sleep on her own at bedtime?

First, reevaluate what is happening at bedtime. Are there any remnants of negative sleep associations that are causing her to have continued difficulties putting herself back to sleep when she wakes during the night? What is it that your child still needs from you during the night? If it is something that is also happening at bedtime, change your bedtime plan and see if that works. If there seems to be no connection between what happens at bedtime and what you need to do in the middle of the night, you will have to do the checking routine during the night. When you go in to check on her, stay for a brief time, no more than one minute, and keep your contact neutral. Don't pick her up. Calmly remind her that it is time to sleep. As with the basic bedtime method, feel free to check as frequently or infrequently as you wish. If your baby still wants a bottle during the night or wants to nurse, then use the method outlined in Chapter 6, decreasing the number of ounces in the bottle over time or the number of minutes you nurse.

Other children continue to wake up during the night as a result of mixed messages. For example, you may decide that if your child wakes up after 4:00 or 5:00 or whatever time you have arbitrarily chosen, you will feed her or bring her to bed with you. Realize that your child can't tell time. To her this is being inconsistent. From her point of view, sometimes you feed her or bring her to your bed, whereas other times you don't. To help your child learn to self-soothe to sleep, you will need to be totally consistent. Wait until it is light out before getting her up for the day and feeding her.

If your child still wakes during the night and doesn't need you anymore to help her get back to sleep, you may want to consider whether your child may be experiencing another type of sleep problem. For example, if she is waking and screaming inconsolably for a period of time, eventually falling back to sleep, she may be having night terrors. If she wakes coughing and choking, she may be suffering from sleep apnea. These and other common sleep disorders are covered in Chapters 12, 13, and 14.

WAKES UP AFTER AN HOUR

Early during sleep training, many babies wake up just an hour after falling asleep at bedtime. Because of sleep deprivation, which may result from your baby doing sleep training and thus falling asleep later than usual, your baby will wake more often (not less, as you would expect). So this may just be an early nighttime awakening. Also, this may be a sleep terror (see Chapter 13), again a result of sleep deprivation. If it is a sleep terror, the best thing is to do as little as possible. Touching your child, or even just saying her name, can make the crying worse and make it last longer.

Don't worry about these one-hour-later awakenings too much. Within a week or two of your baby falling asleep more quickly at bedtime, these awakenings will likely resolve on their own. If they continue, treat them as nighttime awakenings (see above).

TWO PARENTS, TWO REACTIONS

A common scenario in sleep training is that a child will respond differently to each parent. Your child may go to bed great for Dad but not for Mom (or vice versa). This is very common. Children respond differently for many reasons. One parent may be known as the pushover, whereas the other parent is stricter in setting limits. For example, perhaps Daddy will usually give in and read an extra story, whereas Mommy won't. Also, your child may simply be in a stage of preferring one parent over another (most children go through stages of preferring one parent over another, and her choice of preferred parent will change over time). There are several options for dealing with this issue.

+ **Synchronize.** One way to help resolve this issue is to synchronize what you do. Sit down and talk through what each of you does at bedtime. Agree on a similar bedtime routine and similar steps that each of you will take.
+ **Be consistent.** If one parent is adamant about no extra stories, then the other should do the same. If one parent never lies down with their toddler in the middle of the night, then neither should the other parent. Establishing consistent rules will take some compromise.
+ **One parent only.** If your little one always does much better for one parent than the other, put that parent on bedtime or nighttime duty for a week or two. Once things have settled into a better pattern, slowly reintroduce the other parent.

THE EARLY RISER

One common parental complaint is that their child wakes too early in the morning. And while getting up early in the morning is part of being a parent, getting up with your child at 5:00 in the morning is stretching it for most people.

There are two groups of children who wake early in the morning. The first group is those who wake up before they get enough sleep. The second group is those who get enough sleep, and their normal waking time is early in the morning.

Waking Too Early Without Getting Enough Sleep

Some children wake up early in the morning before completing their last sleep cycle. Since there are many transitions in sleep in the early-morning hours, many things can fully awaken your child. For instance, something in your child's environment may be causing the problem, such as early sunlight or the sound of someone getting up to go to work. Being hungry or having a wet diaper can also awaken your child. For other children, this early-morning awakening is just a last night waking. The problem is that children who require their parents to be present to fall asleep at bedtime may require this attention to return to sleep early in the morning.

One way to tell if your child is waking before getting enough sleep is to look at her behavior. Does she seem more sleepy than usual? Does she return to sleep an hour or two after her early-morning rising? Remember, it is rare for an infant or toddler to need less than nine or ten hours of sleep per night. So if your child is waking after less than ten hours of sleep, look for reasons.

+ **Environmental reasons.** If something in your child's environment is waking her or keeping her awake after a natural awakening, remedy the situation. Install room-darkening shades in her bedroom if the sunlight is streaming in at 5:00 in the morning. If there is too much noise from the garbage trucks going by in the morning, try to dampen the noise with a fan or anything else that makes a constant noise.
+ **Wet diaper.** A wet diaper can be resolved by double-diapering or putting your child in superabsorbent diapers made for nighttime. The extra expense of these types of

diapers is well worth the better night's sleep. Also, if your child is drinking a great deal throughout the night, try cutting back on these liquids.

✦ **Behavioral issue.** If your child is waking early in the morning, only to return to sleep quickly, resolving a poor sleep association as outlined in Chapter 6 will get her sleeping until a more reasonable hour. You'll likely need to do sleep training at 5:00 in the morning, similar to the basic bedtime method (presented on page 100). Also, see the prior section in this chapter on dealing with continued night wakings.

✦ **Move bedtime earlier.** Surprisingly, often moving bedtime earlier will solve the problem of the early riser. This suggestion sounds counterintuitive, but it really works. When a child is sleep deprived, he'll wake more often rather than less often. In addition, once a child wakes at 5:00 or 6:00 in the morning, he may have slept enough to make it hard to return to sleep. If you move bedtime earlier, he'll wake less often and be more likely to sleep through the early-morning awakening. Try it. The worst that can happen is that your child will still get up too early, but he'll have gotten more sleep. It's highly unlikely that he'll wake up even earlier.

✦ **"Good-morning light."** Some families have found using a "good-morning light" to be very helpful. A good-morning light is a light that turns on in the morning and lets your child know that it is time to get up for the day (this method works best with older toddlers). The easiest thing to do is to attach a night-light to a timer (the kind that you use to set lamps to turn on and off when you are on vacation). Set the timer for a reasonable time. At first, this time may be earlier than you wish. You can gradually move it later. Explain to your child that when the light is on, then she can get up for the day. When the light is off, then it's still night-night time. You can do something similar with an alarm clock that is set to play music at a certain time. The advantage of the night-light is that it won't wake your child if she's still sleeping. It will likely take a little while before your child understands the concept of a morning signal.

The Early Riser Who Has Had Enough Sleep

Lacey, age two, is in bed and asleep by 7:30 every night. Unfortunately for her parents, she is up and ready to face the day by 6:00 in the morning.

Some children who are up and raring to go early in the morning have gotten a full night's sleep by 5:30 or 6:00 in the morning. Typically, these early birds go to bed by 7:00 or 7:30 in the evening. This is good for the parents because it frees them for activities at night, but it takes away their ability to sleep later in the morning. Your child can sleep only so much. With these children, choose what works best for you: an early bedtime or a later wake time in the morning.

Children can also learn that just because they are up, it doesn't mean that others must get up too. Children need to learn to respect the fact that others may be asleep when they are awake. Parents can establish a clear signal as to when it is okay to start the day. A clock radio can help solve this problem. When the alarm goes off and your child hears the music, that signals when everyone can get up. Before that, she must play quietly without waking the rest of the family.

Parents should also decide what their child is allowed to do in the morning before everyone else is awake. If you allow your child to be up early, make sure that he does not have access to anyplace where he can get hurt and that he is unable to let himself out of the house to play outdoors. Determine whether he is allowed to watch television or turn on a video. A special place for morning toys, such as books and puzzles, can be set up. Add a bowl of cereal if your child is usually hungry first thing in the morning. For younger children, busy boxes and toys in the crib can help entertain them. You can even put several toys in your child's crib once he is asleep that he can play with once he wakes in the morning. You cannot expect him to stay quiet without something to amuse him.

Mary and Roger solved this problem with their early riser, Nathan. By the time he turned three, they had taught Nathan how to turn on the heat in winter months, get out a bowl of Cheerios that they had left for him downstairs, and look through books. In the morning when they got up, they would find him happily ensconced on his favorite stool next to the heat vent in the kitchen, munching on Cheerios and "reading" to himself.

If your child cannot be left without supervision, someone is going to have to get up when he gets up. If you have a partner, negotiate taking turns with this early-morning duty so that each of you gets to sleep in sometimes.

THE NIGHT OWL

In contrast to parents of early risers, there are some parents whose major concern is that their child goes to bed too late at night. These night owls are perfectly content to stay awake until 10:00 or 11:00 at night, and sleep until 9:00 in the morning. If they are put to bed earlier in the evening, these children will toss and turn, unable to fall asleep until their usual later bedtime. On mornings that they need to get up early, they will be difficult to waken. Night owls are not resistant to bedtime; they just are not sleepy or ready to go to bed until a much later hour.

You cannot simply move a night owl's bedtime to an earlier hour. If you put your child in bed at 7:30 when he is unable to fall asleep until 10:30, he will lie awake for three hours. Thus, he will not associate his bed with sleep but rather with being awake and bored. To move a night owl's bedtime earlier, you will need to do it gradually. Start with the time when your child normally falls asleep as your first bedtime. For the next three nights, put your child to bed at this bedtime. Your child should fall asleep easily and quickly. Next, move the bedtime earlier by fifteen minutes, and wake your child fifteen minutes earlier in the morning. After three nights, move bedtime and wake time earlier again by fifteen minutes. Continue this pattern of moving your child's bedtime and wake time earlier by fifteen minutes every three nights until you reach the desired bedtime. With children who can't tell time, moving bedtime earlier in a gradual fashion will not lead to any resistance. They won't even know they are going to bed earlier.

Stanley was successful at moving his two-year-old son's bedtime to an earlier time by using this gradual approach. Previously, Charles was not going to bed until 11:00 at night. After three nights, Stanley moved Charles's bedtime to 10:45. Three nights later, bedtime was 10:30. After several weeks, Charles was going to bed at 8:30 at night, and Stanley and his wife were finally able to have some time to themselves. They also found that Charles was happier in the morning, and he did not resist getting dressed or eating breakfast.

Basically, the time when a child falls asleep at night is determined by the time when he wakes up in the morning (or wakes up from a nap). So to keep a night owl on track, you need to be sure to get him up early in the morning. Bright light in the morning will also help set a child's clock for the day. So head out for a stroll or to a play-ground in the morning, or at least spend time in a sunny part of the house first thing in the morning.

TWINS . . . OR MORE

Twins can be twice as much fun and twice as much work. Sleep problems with twins can also be twice as difficult, especially since each baby will have his or her own idiosyncratic sleep issues. And one twin invariably seems to wake the other. Take twin issues one step further if you have triplets or more.

One of the most frequent questions asked by parents of twins is whether or not to have the twins share a room. Most parents opt to keep them together. If multiple babies start sleeping in the same room from the very beginning, they rarely wake each other up. They will learn to tune each other out. So if one starts fussing, don't take her to another room. The other twin will likely sleep until he is ready to get up.

Another commonly asked question is whether to put them on the same sleep schedule. The answer is a resounding *yes!* It is best to enforce simultaneous naptimes and bedtimes. The babies will do better being on a schedule, and more important, you need the quiet time to energize yourself for when they are both up.

From early on, put twins or triplets down to sleep when they are awake. As with single babies, twins need to learn from an early age to fall asleep on their own and to be self-soothers. Since there is more than one of them, there will often be times when they will need to soothe themselves and be patient. You have only one lap and two hands. Even with two adults, twins are a handful. As diffi-cult as it may seem, try to schedule all sleep times and all naps to-gether. Give yourself plenty of time to get both of them changed and ready for bed before putting them down to sleep. The risk with twins or triplets is that while you are busy with one, the other one will fall asleep in a swing or a high chair. You don't want this to happen. Even though she fell asleep on her own, she needs to do it in the right place: the crib.

Dealing with twins becomes even more interesting when they reach the age of six to nine months. That is when they discover their built-in playmate. Before, you had worried that one's crying would wake the other. Now it is the fun and laughing that you need to worry about. Discourage twins from waking up and playing together during the night or in the early hours of the morning. One trick that Sylvia used with Gregory and Matthew was to place a quiet toy in each of their cribs once they were both asleep. This way when one woke up in the morning, he would have a quiet toy to play with without waking the other. Stuffed animals and busy box–type toys are good choices.

Parents often wonder how to deal with doing sleep training when there are multiples, especially if only one child has sleep problems. You have two choices. One choice is to do sleep training while keeping both children in their cribs or beds. Surprisingly, it works. You may have a few bad nights when one wakes the other, but in the long run you will solve the problem. Another choice is to move out the good sleeper for a few nights while doing sleep training.

As your twins or triplets get older, another problem that is multiplied is their getting out of the crib. One child getting out of a crib is bad enough; two can be dangerous. With two there is a higher likelihood of someone's getting hurt because they are more likely to try to get into things that they shouldn't. Also, an unsupervised aggressive toddler can be a serious danger to another toddler. Be firm in your rules that no one is allowed out of his crib without permission. Install crib tents early on. You may also want to keep twins in their cribs as long as possible to contain their antics.

SHARING A ROOM

Many children share a room with a brother or sister or with someone else in the household. There is often concern that the two people sharing a room will wake each other. Surprisingly, this rarely happens. After a few weeks of sharing, most individuals, children included, rarely are awakened by the other person.

In some situations, though, the child with a sleep problem will disrupt the person sharing his or her room. In these cases, creative solutions are necessary. One solution is to move the sibling out of the room until the child with the sleep problem is sleeping through the night. In a full-force effort, this should take only one to two weeks. Another possibility is to begin sleep training at other times of the day, such as at naptime. In this way the process will not disrupt the other person's sleep.

Jim was seventeen months old and shared a room with his older brother, Michael, who was three. At bedtime, Felicia would get Michael ready for bed and tuck him in. Then she would turn the lights off and rock Jim to sleep. Throughout the night when Jim would wake, Felicia would take him out of his crib and rock him back to sleep. The few times that she didn't, Jim's cries woke Michael. On a few nights she put Jim down in his crib awake. He cried so much that it upset Michael, so she gave up. After months of getting little sleep, however, Felicia was at her wits' end. Her solution was to spend a week putting Jim down for his naps awake in his crib. He was very upset for the first three days, but by the end of the week he was falling asleep quickly. She was then ready to start bedtime training. The first two nights she put Michael to sleep in her bed. Since this was a special treat, Michael thought it was great. She then put Jim in his crib awake. The first night was difficult, but Jim had gotten the message from naptime training. Once Jim was asleep, she moved Michael back into his own bed. On the third night both boys were put to bed in their room. Jim was fussy, but Felicia was surprised to hear Michael telling Jim that it was okay and to go to sleep—the exact words that she had used!

SINGLE PARENTS

As a single parent, there are times when you are going to need help. Face it: parenting is hard enough in two-parent families, but when it is only you—and especially if you have more than one child—it can easily become overwhelming. Single parents need even more support from others than do dual parents. A single parent needs a sounding board to help make parenting decisions. Single parents also need downtime. Day after day and night after night of constant child rearing is difficult to do. No matter how much you love your child, you need a break. So figure out ways to get help. Pay a babysitter to watch your child, whether you go out or stay home. A less expensive alternative is to swap child care time with other parents. All parents appreciate the time off. If you know of a group of parents with children of similar ages, establish a babysitting cooperative. A record can be kept of who has given babysitting time and who owes babysitting time. Everyone gets free child care, and everyone gets time off.

Some single parents feel guilty that their child does not have a mother and a father. To compensate for this guilt, some single parents are reluctant to set limits, allowing their child more free rein. This is a recipe for sleep problems. It is often easier for a single parent just to give in: what difference does it make if the child stays up a half hour later or sleeps in the parent's bed just this night?

Well, it does matter. Children need routines and they need to have limits set, whether they have two parents, one parent, or another type of caregiver. So be sure to have a daily routine and set bedtime rules.

APARTMENT LIVING

Families who live in apartments may have more problems teaching their babies to sleep than those living in single homes, because of worries about disturbing the neighbors. It may be virtually impossible to let your baby cry at 2:00 in the morning with neighbors nearby. This is especially true in the summertime, when windows are open. Some parents are concerned that their neighbors might even think that their baby is being abused or neglected because they are letting him cry for such an extended period of time.

If you have these or similar concerns because you live with others or close to others, there are solutions. Remember, the important part of getting your baby to sleep through the night is teaching him to fall asleep on his own. This does not have to happen at one specific time. Rather than teaching your baby to self-soothe at bedtime, do it at naptimes during the week, when most people are gone for the day. You can also choose your days. Begin sleep training on a Friday night so it will disturb only weekend sleep. And by all means warn your neighbors. Explain your predicament and what you are trying to do. Beware, though, that you may be the recipient of lots of unwanted and contradictory advice about how to manage your baby's sleep problems.

Reminders —————————————————————————————

+ Anticipate pitfalls to teaching your child good sleeping habits.
+ Be firm about your child's climbing out of the crib and getting out of bed.

- ✦ Breast-feeding can make sleep issues more complicated.
- ✦ Be prepared to deal with "I have to go potty" and "Just one more hug."
- ✦ Developmental milestones such as rolling over can interfere with your baby's ability to fall asleep.
- ✦ Parents in special circumstances—whether having twins, being a single parent, or living in an apartment—need to anticipate common obstacles to sleeping through the night.
- ✦ No matter what the situation, find solutions that promote positive sleep associations and do not reinforce negative sleep associations.

CHAPTER 11

To Grandma's House We Go:
Changes in Routine and Other Obstacles to
Continued Good Sleep

Kathleen and Brian recently separated. They have joint custody of their three-year-old daughter, Courtney. Courtney spends weekdays with Kathleen and weekends with Brian. Both Kathleen and Brian find that Courtney has difficulty falling asleep on the first night that she sleeps at either's house.

Once a baby is sleeping through the night, parents often feel that the worst is over. While this is true, there may still be obstacles to face, such as vacations, overnights at grandparents', babysitters, special occasions, and times when the baby gets sick. Other common obstacles include managing an older child's sleep after the birth of a new baby or the divorce of parents. Each of these situations, and more, can disrupt your child's sleep.

DEALING WITH BUMPS IN THE ROAD

Ellen's two-year-old son, Nathaniel, finally started sleeping through the night at fourteen months. But for the past few weeks he has

*refused to go to bed and won't sleep in his room. All of these prob-
lems began after the family returned from a summer vacation.*

No matter how well things go with getting your baby to sleep
through the night, there will always be bumps in the road. There
will always be a time when your child has a bad night, whether because she is teething, got sick, spent a night away from home, or for
no apparent reason at all (the hardest one for parents to cope with).
When, all of a sudden, for whatever reason or no apparent reason,
their child suddenly starts waking during the night or having trouble falling asleep at bedtime, many parents respond to these set-
backs by going into sleep crisis mode. They start trying different
things each night, looking for the magical solution. "He must be
hungry"—so they feed him. "He must be upset"—so they take him
downstairs and lie on the couch from 4:00 a.m. on. "He must be going through separation anxiety"—so they take him to their bed.
These actions are done with the best of intentions, but unfortunately
they just confuse the entire process. Instead of changing what you are
doing, you need to be totally consistent and stick with what has
always worked. I always recommend giving the benefit of the doubt
for the first night or two—feed him, stay with him, whatever—but on
the third night, it's become a habit. Just as sleep problems can often
be fixed in three nights, so sleep problems can also be created in three
nights. So try not to go too far astray from your routine on the first
couple of nights, and after that stick to what has always worked—
same bedtime, same bedtime routine, and same nighttime rules.
Otherwise, you'll soon be stuck in a place you never wanted to be—
such as on the living room couch with your baby every night at
4:00 a.m.

VACATIONS

When Becky was eight months old, Francine and George decided to go on vacation—their first since Becky was born. They went to Florida with Becky and stayed with George's parents in a condominium on the beach. Before the vacation, Becky slept great. They put her to bed at 8:00 and wouldn't hear from her again until she woke at 6:30 in the morning. On vacation her sleep began to become problematic. Because his parents' condominium had only two bedrooms, Becky slept in the same room as Francine and George. In addition to sleeping in the same room with her parents and being upset by being in a new place, Becky's sleep schedule was disturbed because they would often stay out late visiting friends or going out to dinner. By the end of the vacation, Francine and George were ready to return home and to their routine. What they didn't expect was that Becky continued to have sleep problems. The first night was difficult because they had an evening flight and therefore did not get home until 11:00 at night. The next morning Becky slept until 9:00, which threw off her nap schedule. Then bedtime became difficult. While Becky used to go right to sleep on her own, now she required someone to hold her until she fell asleep. She was also waking two to three times per night. Francine and George vowed never to go on vacation again until Becky was eighteen!

Vacations are known to disturb babies' sleep schedules. There are a number of reasons for this common problem. Francine and George's story is fairly typical. Often on vacation, parents have the baby sleeping in the room with them. They may also have to respond to their baby during the night because they are concerned about the baby's crying disturbing others in the hotel or house where they are staying. The baby's sleep schedule is often changed because of plans that disrupt normal naptimes and bedtime. There are things to do during the day and places to go in the evening. Babysitters may not be available, so the parents are often forced to bring the baby along with them. Because the baby is sleeping in a strange environment, she may be more inclined to have problems falling asleep at night and difficulties with waking during the night. As a parent you are also much less likely to set limits because you know that it is difficult for the baby to be sleeping in a new place. You yourself may even have problems sleeping in a new place and can sympathize with your baby's sleeplessness. In addition, a change of time zone may wreak havoc on everyone's schedule.

Upon returning home, most parents expect that their baby's sleep will return to normal. It often doesn't. Their baby has quickly become used to being rocked to sleep or at least having them stay with her or respond to her during the night. She may also be used to sleeping in the same room with them, something she may thoroughly enjoy whether they did or not.

Never going on vacation again is not the best solution. There are things that you can do to minimize sleep problems associated with vacations. The key to sleeping through the night on vacations is to make things as similar to home as possible. Here are some suggestions.

ROOM ARRANGEMENTS. If possible, if you don't share a room with your baby at home, try not to share a room with your baby on vacation. Obviously, you may not have a choice. But if you do, opt to have your baby stay in her own room rather than share with you. This will be more like what she is used to and will help ease the transition. If you are concerned about hearing her during the night, bring along a baby monitor. If you can afford it, book a suite at a hotel so that the baby can sleep in a separate space. Another idea is to section off part of the room by hanging a sheet as a partition. Walk-in closets can also easily be converted into a second bedroom for a portable crib. Some hotel rooms have separate sitting areas, a less expensive option than a suite or two rooms. Staying at a small inn or bed-and-breakfast may also help. This way, in the evenings, you can be in the sitting room enjoying the fire and a book, or having a late dinner in the inn's restaurant, while your baby is in your room asleep. Be sure to bring along your baby monitor so you can hear what is going on with your baby. (And prior to making the reservations, confirm that babies are allowed at the inn.)

BEDDING AND FAVORITE ITEMS. Bring your baby's blanket or other bedding with you. This may be inconvenient to carry, especially if you are traveling by plane, but you'll find it truly worthwhile. Your baby will sleep better in her own familiar bedding. The smell, feel, and texture will help soothe her. Also, if your baby sleeps with a favorite stuffed animal or other item, be absolutely sure that you do not forget it. Many a family has had to turn the car around halfway to their destination because they forgot "bunny" or "teddy."

SLEEP SCHEDULES. Although this can be difficult while on vacation, try to keep sleep schedules as similar as possible to your baby's schedule at home. Try to keep all naptimes and bedtimes the same. Although this may interfere with your vacation plans, you will be happier with a baby who is not cranky and overtired. This may require hiring a babysitter or splitting baby duty with your spouse. One of you may need to stay with the baby while the other goes off to play. Switch off baby duty so that everyone has time for fun. Yes, vacations will be different from what you were used to, but adjusting to a baby requires certain changes.

CHANGING TIME ZONES. Babies are just as likely as adults to experience jet lag. If you are staying only one to three days, it's best to try and stay on your home schedule. Any longer, though, and you'll need to adjust to the new time zone. There are several things that you can try. First of all, try to choose flights that allow you to land in the late afternoon or early evening. Then stay awake until it is bedtime. In the morning, be sure to wake your baby at the time she normally wakes up. Keep naps on schedule too. Also, be sure to get your baby out into daylight. Different times of the day are best for exposure to sunlight to reset the body clock, depending on whether you are traveling east or west and how many time zones you are crossing. You can find jet lag calculators on several online Web sites to help figure out what is the best time of day to get out in bright light.

BEDTIME ROUTINE. Ideally, you have established a bedtime routine at home. Keep to the same routine on vacation. If your baby's routine is to take a bath, put on pajamas, read a book, and sing a song, then by all means while on vacation bathe, change, read, and sing away. Since everything is so new on vacation, your baby will appreciate some familiar routines.

TRAVEL SCHEDULES. When making travel arrangements, keep your baby's sleep schedule in mind. If you are taking a two-hour car ride or train trip, do it when your baby usually naps. This way your baby will sleep on the ride and will be right on schedule when you reach your destination. If you are flying, travel during the day— again, if possible, during usual naptimes. Try to avoid red-eye or late-evening flights, which will force your baby's bedtime to be several hours later than usual. You may not have much choice, of course, if you are traveling a long distance.

RETURNING HOME. The key to getting sleep back to normal is to return immediately to your usual routines the moment you get home. Go through your baby's usual bedtime routine and put her down awake at her usual time. Don't stay with her "just this once" if you usually don't. If you do, she is going to assume that new rules apply, and you will have a battle on your hands. If you go back to the typical home mode right from the start, she will understand that even though things may have been different when you were away, home sleep rules still apply. Of course, your baby may take a night or two to adjust to being back home, but be assured that she will go back to sleeping through the night (that is, if she slept through the night before).

OVERNIGHTS

Staying overnight at someone else's house or at a hotel can be a challenge. Many adults have difficulty sleeping in new places, so don't be surprised if your child has problems too. On the other hand, to many parents' frustration, their child may sleep better at someone else's house. This is usually true only if neither parent is present.

———

Lorraine's baby, Timmy, would never go to sleep in his crib but always insisted on being rocked. He would usually wake two to three times every night, usually between 2:00 and 4:00 in the morning. Whenever Timmy stayed at his grandparents', though, he would go to sleep easily and sleep through the night. As you can imagine, Lorraine wondered if she was doing something wrong, and she found Timmy's sleep problems even more frustrating at home, since she knew he really could sleep through the night.

———

Your child may sleep better for others because he does not have the ingrained sleep associations elsewhere that he has with you. If your child needs you to nurse or rock him to sleep, he has to figure out some other way to soothe himself to sleep when you are not available. Take this as a good sign. It means that your child has the ability to comfort himself and put himself to sleep. You just need to train him to do this in his own home.

For babies who have problems sleeping at other places, there are a few things that you can do. First, make sure that your child has familiar items with him. Send along his favorite blanket or stuffed animal. Tell the person with whom he is staying about his usual routine. If you are with him at someone else's house, take your time and don't scrimp on his bedtime routine. Your baby will sense if you are rushing him, and you will pay the price when he resists going to bed. No matter how well or poorly it goes when your child is sleeping someplace else other than home, return immediately to your usual routine when you get back home. Don't build in a "transition night." This will only confuse your child. You need to help your child learn that certain limits consistently apply when at home. Just one night of giving in and staying with him until he falls asleep will limit your ability to follow through on subsequent nights.

Remember, it is important for your child to be able to sleep at other places. Just because he has a difficult time sleeping elsewhere and then has problems making the transition to being home doesn't mean that you should give up and never let him stay anywhere other than home. He just needs some practice, and after several times of dealing with the transition, things will start to go more smoothly.

BABYSITTERS

For the past two weeks you have been working diligently at getting your baby to go to sleep without fussing, and he is finally sleeping through the night for the first time in eight months. This coming Saturday night, however, you have to be at a family event, and so you have a babysitter coming over. You are worried that she'll have a struggle getting your baby to sleep, all of your hard work will have been wasted, and you will end up right back where you started. What should you do?

The best thing to do is to be prepared. Although your child may be sleeping great for you, the first night with someone different putting him to bed can be difficult. Remember that even if your child has problems sleeping when a babysitter is caring for him, he will return to sleeping well for you. It may take a little practice, though, for your child to understand the difference between your rules and a babysitter's rules. Instead of worrying about that, try to prevent that type of situation from occurring. If this is your usual babysitter, have the person arrive early. Explain what you have been doing and about your child's new sleeping habits. Give the babysitter step-by-step instructions on your child's new bedtime routine. Inform the babysitter that your child is to be put to bed awake; tell him or her what to say, when to leave the room, and what to do if your child fusses or cries. Explain that you realize this may be difficult and discuss how to cope with the baby's crying. Explain thoroughly why you are doing this and why it is important.

If you're using a paid babysitter, you shouldn't have too many problems getting him or her to implement your instructions. If the babysitter is a family member, especially a grandparent, it may be more difficult. Family members are much more likely to express their opinion on this process and may not like what you are doing: "How can I let my grandchild cry? It is so cruel." You have two choices in this situation. Choice one is to explain the process and emphasize the positive strides that have been made. The other choice is to leave it alone. Your child will still go to sleep for you as long as you are consistent, although it may take a night or two to readjust to your new rules after a pushover night with Grandma and Grandpa. Also, once your child is going to sleep easily, the grandparents will see the change and want things to go as smoothly. Your baby will also get to the point of insisting on his usual bedtime routine so that he can fall asleep. Good sleep associations are just as hard to break as bad ones.

SPECIAL OCCASIONS

One of the things that seem to go along with special occasions is staying up later at night. Whether it is a birthday celebration, the Fourth of July, or another holiday, children often stay up late and miss out on their bedtime routines. They also may stay up late, fall asleep on the car ride home, and then get put to bed already asleep.

When your child stays up late, he may become overtired and cranky. This can make settling him down for bed more difficult. Don't forsake a bedtime routine because it is late. You may want to shorten it a bit, reading one story instead of two, for example, but don't eliminate it entirely. Your child needs his routine to fall asleep and sleep through the night. Without a routine, you may pay the price with a middle-of-the-night waking. Also, don't try to rush your child. It will just unsettle him and can make the entire process take longer if he balks at being rushed.

What should you do if your child has been out late somewhere other than home and falls asleep before getting home? Some parents find that their child will sleep better if they wake him after getting home and do at least a part of the bedtime routine. Your child may not want to wake up and may be a bit crabby, but it can help the transition. It will also make it easier for your child when he wakes up in the middle of the night and finds himself in his bed at home when the last thing he remembers is being in the car. There is no need to wake an infant, but it can be beneficial for a child over the age of one. For some children, however, waking them causes more problems because they will be overtired and cranky, and then will stay awake for a long time before settling back down again. It will take some experimentation to see what works best for your child.

ILLNESS

Sharleena, eight months, has frequent ear infections. Whenever she gets an infection, she starts having trouble falling asleep at night and wakes frequently throughout the night. Since Sharleena is so young, her parents sometimes have a hard time determining when the ear infection has cleared up and whether Sharleena is just waking from habit rather than from any ear discomfort.

Illness always wreaks havoc on sleep. During an illness your baby will most likely have a difficult time falling asleep, will wake frequently throughout the night, and will probably be cranky on top of everything else. Then, once sleep patterns get thrown off, it will take a while to return to normal. And it is often hard to tell when the illness is over and your baby is again feeling fine.

When your baby is sick, you have no choice but to go to her during the night when she wakes up. She doesn't feel well and may be in pain. She is going to need soothing. If you typically do not let your child sleep with you, try to avoid bringing her to your bed when she is not feeling well. Often, it is better to sleep in her room than to bring her to yours. This way she will have the comfort of her own bed and you will be nearby. A futon, an inflatable mattress, or just a pile of blankets on the floor will make your night a bit more comfortable. It is much better to go stay with your child, where she is most comfortable, than to bring her to you. You may have an uncomfortable night or two, but your little one will stay snug in her own bed.

Once you are sure that she is well again, go right back to your normal bedtime routine and return to setting limits on her behavior during the night. After several bouts with ear infections or colds, she will begin to understand the rule: when not sick, bedtime rules apply. If you are in the midst of sleep training or have just finally gotten your child sleeping through the night, don't despair. Once well again, your child will quickly resume the progress that she has made.

Don't be surprised if your baby has sleep problems if she is often sick. Research has shown that babies who are often sick or who are colicky are the least likely to sleep through the night. But don't despair; you are not alone.

TEETHING

Parents often comment that their baby was sleeping fine until he began to teethe. Surprisingly, however, teething is probably not the main cause of sleep problems. First teeth usually begin to come in sometime between six months and ten months. Although teething may cause some problems with sleep, it is more likely that it is coincidence. Studies have shown that sleep problems increase at this age and are related to normal development. Babies continue to get teeth until the age of two or two and a half. But most babies do not continue to have problems sleeping, supporting the contention that there is little relationship between teething and sleep problems. But if your baby is having some problems sleeping when teething, there are some things to try.

Babies will be fussy when they are teething. It does not feel good. They will drool more and want to bite on things. Provide your baby with lots of soft things to chew on. There are teething toys specifically made to ease teething pain. Most are placed in the refrigerator or freezer. The coldness helps soothe the baby's gums. Children's Tylenol can also be helpful, but be sure to check with your pediatrician before giving your baby any medication.

If your baby is having sleeping problems at the same time he is teething, be sure that he doesn't have a fever or other symptoms of illness. If all seems fine except for the teething, be consistent about sleep issues. Even a few nights of changing the rules can lead to many a sleepless night for you and your baby.

DEVELOPMENTAL MILESTONES

Developmental milestones are notorious for disrupting your child's sleep. Whether you are just starting sleep training or have had a great sleeper for months, developmental milestones are likely to disrupt your baby's sleep. Not only will the milestone itself affect your baby's sleep, but many parents report that their baby's sleep seems to fall apart the couple of weeks before a major change. Obviously, you won't know it's coming, but don't be surprised if a week after your baby starts waking up again at night, she all of a sudden figures out how to crawl or walk. A recent study documented this relationship. Babies were found to have a harder time settling down to sleep and to be waking more at night the two weeks before they took their first steps. Also, realize that for your baby it's much more fun to practice crawling or pulling to standing than it is to sleep. In most cases, you'll need to wait until the novelty wears off. While you are waiting, stick to what you always do in terms of your bedtime routine and how you respond to your baby during the night. You don't want to create a longer-term problem.

Rolling Over

Melissa's daughter, Sally, is five months old and has learned how to roll from her back to her stomach but can't roll the other way yet. She sleeps on her back, so once she rolls onto her stomach, she can't turn over and needs someone to flip her back. This happens at least twice during the night.

At some point, your baby may roll over and not be able to roll back. This is a problem if she can fall asleep only on one side. If it is sleep time, the minute she rolls over onto her stomach she will cry for you to turn her back over. This may continue to happen throughout the night. There is not much you can do about this other than to go in and turn the baby over. You may try to teach your baby to roll back the other way, but you can't really speed up motor development in a baby this young. Once you are sure, though, that she can roll back, leave her to figure it out on her own.

By five or six months, most babies are able to roll themselves from their backs, so if you were putting your baby to sleep on her back as recommended, you have now lost control of keeping her there. Many parents become quite concerned about this because of the risk of SIDS. Once a baby can roll over from her back, she is usually past the risk of SIDS. There is no need to spend all night worrying and going in to turn your baby back over. Check with your pediatrician, though, who can assess your baby's risk for SIDS. Also, don't try restricting her movement by swaddling her or putting her in clothes in which she is unable to move around. This is not a solution to the problem of her rolling over.

Standing Up in the Crib

Bruce's seven-and-a-half-month-old son, Ian, has a new trick. After Bruce puts him to bed and leaves the room, Ian pulls himself up, stands there holding on to the railing, and cries. The problem is that Ian can't get back down. It has been going on for days!

Some babies begin to pull themselves up to standing as early as five months, whereas others may not do so until they are a year old. In either case, these babies often have a difficult time sitting back down. Stranded, they become frustrated and begin to cry, waiting for someone to help them down, or they simply collapse. Once helped down, they invariably pull themselves back up immediately and get stuck again. This can become tedious and frustrating for parents.

When your baby begins to pull herself up to standing, help her down slowly and gently so that she learns how to do it herself. This learning process should take only a few days, although some babies may take a few weeks to learn this new skill. In the beginning you will have no choice but to rescue her. If your baby is doing this at naptime and bedtime, go in and, in a neutral manner, help her sit or lie down. If you get too involved, she will keep standing up and crying to get your attention. During the day, at times other than bedtime, have her practice pulling up and sitting back down. Once you are sure that she has the ability to sit back down, stop rescuing her when she is in her crib or it will become a game to her.

Also, be sure to safety-proof your baby's crib. Don't leave any hard objects, such as busy boxes, on which she can bang her head if she falls.

TOILET TRAINING

"I have to go potty!" is a statement that few parents can ignore. And young children quickly learn that when toilet training begins, "going potty" takes precedence over almost anything else. The moment that you get a child all bundled up into a snowsuit, the child will declare that she has to go potty. The moment that you are a mile from your home and are late for an appointment, your toddler will claim a desperate need to go potty. The same thing happens at sleep times: the moment your toddler is settled into her crib or bed, she will insist that she needs to go to the bathroom, even if she just went.

There are two ways to deal with this situation. The first is to make sure that your child always goes to the bathroom before going down for a nap or to bed for the night. The second way is to allow your child one extra time going to the bathroom. Plan for this and expect it to happen, so you won't get frustrated when she claims the need to go. When she does call out, get her and take her to the bathroom or give her permission to go on her own. This latter method is also good practice because she will learn what to do when she is in bed and really does need to go to the bathroom. The novelty of trying this tactic at bedtime will soon wear off. (Remember, at the beginning of toilet training, going to the bathroom is a novel and exciting thing to do.) After the first time (or second time if you decide this is reasonable), don't allow any more trips to the bathroom. If you make this rule, be firm and follow through. You should therefore make a decision as to how you are going to handle the call for the potty, and stick to it.

SWITCHING TO A BED

One obstacle that all parents face is how to manage the change from a crib to a bed. The two major questions that arise are "when?" and "how?"

When Do You Make the Switch?

There is no set time that you should get rid of your child's crib and switch to a bed, although most children make the move sometime between one and a half and three and a half years. It is highly recommended that you wait as long as you can. Many children are not developmentally ready until they are closer to three years of age. A crib has clearly defined sides. A bed, however, requires that children understand that there are imaginary boundaries (the edge of the bed) that they must stay within. This understanding requires a high level of cognitive development. Second, it is just not safe for a very young child to be able to be up and about in the middle of the night. A crib is much safer, as a child cannot wander about his room or the house at 2:00 in the morning when everyone else is asleep. Third, for many children, their crib is their special snug place in the world. A change to a bed may seem like a step forward and "better" than a crib to you, but for a young child it may just be the opposite. This change can result in a great sleeper becoming a poor sleeper if the move is made too early.

Many things can trigger the exact time for a change from a crib to a bed. The most common time is prior to the birth of another baby. If this is the reason, you may want to make the switch at least six to eight weeks before your next child is due. You want your older child well settled in his new bed before he sees the new baby taking over his crib. An alternative is not to make the switch until the new baby is three or four months old. Before that time, the newborn may be sleeping in a bassinet anyway. Then, by waiting, your older child will have adjusted to the new baby, making the transition from crib to bed easier.

The second most common reason to make the switch is that your child tries to climb or jump out of the crib. Many parents become concerned about their child's harming himself. This may or may not be a good time to switch to a bed. On the positive side, you will not have to worry about your child's hurting himself in the middle of the night by falling from the crib. On the negative side, switching to a bed does not remove the concerns about your child being able to get up and move about during the night without your knowing it. You will also have lost all control of detaining your child during the night. If your child is very young and you would rather not move him to a bed, strategies for handling the issue of getting out of the crib are given in Chapter 10. You can also simply keep the side of the crib down so that your child can easily get out without having to switch to a bed.

Another reason that many parents decide to make the move to a bed is that their child is in the midst of being potty trained or is already potty trained. While your child is being potty trained, you will want him to be able to get to the bathroom when necessary. Being in a crib may make this impossible. One solution, though, as mentioned previously, is to lower the side of the crib (or remove it entirely) and put a stool by the side of the crib. This allows your child to climb out whenever necessary but still allows him to continue sleeping in a crib. If this sounds dangerous, or you are not sure if your child can handle it, do some test trials and have your child practice. Remember that he may already be climbing up on counters or onto high objects where you don't want him to be, so the climb from the crib may be relatively easy.

Parents sometimes decide to switch their child to a bed because it seems like the right time or their child appears to be outgrowing the crib. Other signs include your little one asking for a bed or your child sleeping well in a bed elsewhere, such as when on vacation or when sleeping at a grandparent's house. These are good reasons to make the move.

A bad reason to make the move is making the change because of pressure from others. Don't worry about it if your mother-in-law tells you that all of her children were in a bed by the time they were two. Honestly, who cares? Instead, do what is right for your child and for your family.

How Do You Make the Switch?

For some children the transition from crib to bed goes smoothly. For others it is more difficult. It usually goes more smoothly than the parents expect, however. One of the most creative ideas that I have heard was from a parent who threw a "big boy's bed" party for her three-year-old. She took him with her to the store to choose the bed, then talked it up for a week in advance. On the day of the big event, she had a party and invited friends and grandparents. There was a cake and balloons. He was so excited about getting a big boy's bed that everything went smoothly.

But while many children relish the move, others are resistant. Each child is different. Your first child is the most likely to resist the transition. He may be very attached to his crib, and it is likely that the switch will be made around the time that a new baby is coming. Switching to sleeping in a bed is one of the many changes that will occur in his life, such as no longer being the baby of the family and the center of attention. It may also coincide with toilet training, another pressure for him to "grow up." Later-born children often make the transition more easily because they want to be just like their older brother or sister. Since their older sibling sleeps in a bed, they will also want to sleep in a bed. To a younger child, a crib may be for "babies."

On your child's first night in the new bed, be sure to follow your child's normal bedtime routine. Read the same number of stories, or sing the usual songs. If you didn't stay with your child until he was asleep when he was in a crib, don't start staying now. Some parents make the mistake of lying down with their child on the first night of the arrival of a big bed. Don't start the habit unless you want to be doing it for a long time. Instead, establish a bedtime routine on the first night exactly the way you want to keep doing it.

Also, don't tell your child *not* to get out of bed. Surprisingly, most children stay put, so don't put the idea in your child's head. If he does get out, matter-of-factly return him to his bed and remind him that it is night-night time. Give him attention for staying in bed, not for getting out.

Should you leave the crib still standing? This is a difficult question to answer. It really depends on your child. The usual suggestion is to take the crib down when you put up the bed. Some people have no choice because they have no room to do otherwise. But even if you have the room, leaving the crib standing may cause difficulty for your child. He may become ambivalent about where he wants to sleep, and the choice may put even more pressure on him during this potentially stressful time. Even if you are expecting another child within a few weeks, you may want to take the crib down for this short time, until your child no longer recognizes it as his and as the place where he sleeps. If you do take the crib down, put the new bed in the same place as the crib to avoid additional changes for your child. Your child also may find it soothing to continue to sleep with his old crib blanket even if it is too small for the bed. Some children, though, are completely ready to move to a bed and will relish this change in their status.

No matter how prepared your child may be to move to a bed, you should always put up a guardrail to prevent him from falling out of the new bed. Some children may resist having the guardrail up at bedtime. Jessica moved into a "big girl's bed" at the age of three. Two months later she insisted that her mother not put the guardrail up at bedtime even though she had fallen out of bed several times when it had been left down. Rather than fight about it, her mother simply left it down at bedtime. After Jessica had fallen asleep, her mother went back in and put it up. This ensured that Jessica was safe but also stopped the arguments at bedtime. Jessica did catch on eventually, but by that time her mother had decided to take the guardrail off the bed completely. Jessica was more accustomed to sleeping in a bed by then and didn't need the guardrail.

In the beginning, after your child has moved to a bed, be alert when your child sleeps in beds other than her own, such as at others' houses or while on vacation. Put up a bed rail or construct a wall of some type so that she doesn't fall out of the bed. At a minimum, place blankets or pillows on the floor to cushion the fall so she won't be hurt if she does fall. Falling out of bed is even scarier for children who are sleeping in a strange bed. Falling out of bed can also occur at other times.

Sarah's mother couldn't understand why Sarah suddenly began falling out of bed a year after being moved to her bed. Then she realized that after she had rearranged Sarah's bedroom furniture, a different side of the bed was against the wall. Before, Sarah could safely roll to the right because the wall was on her right side. With the new furniture arrangement, the wall was now on her left side. In her sleep she would still roll to the right, thinking it was safe, but instead she now landed on the floor. Sarah's mother put a guardrail back on the bed for a few weeks until Sarah got used to this new arrangement.

What should you do if you make the switch and it ends up being a disaster? This happened to Shianna when she switched her daughter to a bed at twenty-two months. Whereas her daughter had been happily going to bed at 8:00 every night, she now wasn't falling asleep until 10:15 or later, and bedtime had become a battle. If the bed isn't working, put the crib back up! There is absolutely no reason not to. It's not a failure. It's simply not the right time. Most parents wouldn't have any qualms about switching back to diapers after trying "big-girl" underwear for a few days. Rather, be matter-of-fact about switching back, or better yet make a big deal out of it. "Hurray, your crib is back! Isn't that exciting?" Remember, it's all in the presentation.

THE BIRTH OF A NEW BABY

The birth of a new baby can lead to sleep problems in older children. Children will often have a period of adjustment to the presence of a new baby in the house. As one mother said about her twenty-month-old, "I swear, he keeps giving me dagger looks and wants to know when 'she' is going to be returned." Having a new baby disrupts everyone's routine. A new baby and a toddler can be even more difficult. A newborn is demanding, especially for the first few months. At the same time, your older child or children need just as much attention as before. And if you and your newborn stay awake much of the night, you won't have the opportunity to sleep during the day because your older child will be running about.

There are some things that you can do, however, to make the transition easier. First of all, prepare your other children for the arrival of their new baby brother or sister as much as you can. Obviously, this will depend upon the age of your older one(s). Read lots of books about being a big brother or sister. Talk about Mommy being gone for a few days and coming home with a new baby. Talk about the new baby in Mommy's tummy. As you set up the nursery for your new baby, have your older child help. Involve him in the process as much as possible.

When it comes to sleep, there are several things that you can do to make the transition to older sibling easier. Remember, your other child may feel displaced by the new baby in terms of your time and affection. Keep that in mind when your older child starts to act up. Children need lots of attention during this time. You may be thinking, "How in the world am I going to do that?" The easiest way is to get help if you can. Your partner will be even more essential in helping out after the birth of a second or third child than with the first. A helper can be a huge benefit in caring for the newborn. To be honest, a one-week-old baby does not care much who changes her diaper, while a two-year-old will care a great deal about who puts him to bed. To keep your older child sleeping through the night, make sure that you make bedtime and bedtime rituals sacred. Try to get someone else to watch the baby while you spend some quality time with your older one. Read books in peace. Put on pajamas and have some fun with your older child. In the beginning you may not be able to do it all alone, especially if you are not allowed to lift anything, but that is okay. Do as much as you can and have someone else lift him into his crib.

Keep bedtime rules consistent. Obviously, someone else will be taking care of your older child while you are off having the next one. Make sure that you have left instructions on your child's sleep rituals. As much as possible, keep everything the same while you are gone. Your child will be better off.

Once you are back home, your child will test the limits. He'll want to check that you are the same parent as before. If only two requests for extra hugs were allowed at bedtime before, then give only two extra hugs now. Four hugs to try to reassure him will only confuse him and make him more concerned. In his mind something must be really wrong if he is getting away with misbehaving. He wants to be sure that all is the same, and setting limits will be reassuring. It will not upset him more.

Another issue that may come up is whether one child will wake the other in the middle of the night. Usually, the older child wakes the newborn rather than the other way around. If your new baby is waking your older child, though, reassure the older one and put him back to bed as quickly as you can. You don't want to reinforce night wakings. It may take older children a few weeks to get used to the sound of a newborn baby crying in the middle of the night, especially if it results in parental attention, but be assured that this, too, will pass and things will return to normal. Keep the faith and don't get too overwhelmed and discouraged. All will settle in, and eventually everyone will sleep again.

TIME CHANGES AND LONGER DAYS

Your child's usual sleeping patterns may get thrown off when the clocks change. In the spring, the clocks get moved forward. This means that if your child goes to sleep at 7:30, after the time change it will really be 6:30 (according to his internal clock) when you put him down. Your child will probably not be tired and may take a long time to fall asleep. Don't change his bedtime to compensate, or the adjustment will take even longer. Just keep putting him to bed at his usual time, when the clock says 7:30. To help him make the transition more quickly, keep waking him at his normal wake time rather than letting him sleep in to compensate for the lost sleep. He may be cranky from being tired, but this should last only a day or two. Another choice is to start moving bedtime earlier before the actual time change. You can start on Saturday night and move bedtime earlier by thirty minutes; or start on Thursday night by moving bedtime earlier by fifteen minutes on each successive night.

In the fall, the clocks get moved back. What used to be 7:30 is now 8:30 (again, according to your child's internal clock). Bedtime should not be a problem. Your child will be tired and definitely ready to go to bed by his bedtime. The problem parents face in the fall is that their child is now waking too early in the morning. Rather than getting up at 6:30, he will be ready to get up for the day at 5:30. For most children, simply be strict about keeping to usual bedtimes, wake times, and naptimes. Keep your child up at night until the clock says it is time to go to bed. This will help him sleep later in the morning. Some parents find it is best to first make these changes on Saturday night rather than wait until Sunday, a school night. And for those children who quickly get overtired if they don't get to bed on time, try making a slow transition starting on Thursday night. Move your child's bedtime later by fifteen minutes each day. By Sunday night you will be right back on schedule. No matter what approach you take, within a few days to a week, your child will have adjusted to the new time and be back to sleeping to his usual wake time.

Along with the clocks changing, another thing that can affect sleep is longer days and shorter nights during summer months. This is especially true the farther north you live. With longer summer days, it may seem strange to put your child to bed at 7:00 at night while it is still bright and sunny outside. Do it anyway. Your child needs his sleep. If the light seems to be bothering him, get room-darkening shades. Remember, babies are used to sleeping when it is light out. They do it all the time when they nap. If they can sleep at naptime when it is light out, they can sleep at bedtime when it is light out. The theme throughout this book is to be consistent. Be consistent and it will all work out.

GOING BACK TO WORK

Mothers often agonize over returning to work. Mothers may go back to work because they need to, because they want to, or both. No matter what the reason, your return to work may be a difficult and emotionally trying time. One possible result of this change is a disruption of your baby's sleep schedule. If your baby wasn't having sleep problems before, he may begin to have them now. On the other hand, if your baby wasn't sleeping before, the problem will remain the same and may even get worse.

Your baby's sleep schedule is affected by your return to work for several reasons. First of all, your baby's routine changes. Whether he is in day care or is being cared for at home by someone else (even the baby's father), everyone does things slightly differently, and your baby will notice the difference. The timing of his usual naptimes may change, especially if his early-morning schedule is affected by your return to work. He is likely to be put down to sleep in a different way: rather than being nursed or sung to, he may be given a bottle or just cuddled. No matter what, this will be a time of transition for your baby. This is not a bad thing. Babies need to be able to adapt to different environments and different people.

In addition, your behavior will likely change when you return to work simply because of the changes in your life. You are now juggling several roles and multiple demands. You are likely to be more tired. Also, many mothers feel guilty about returning to work and leaving their baby. This guilt may cause you to project your feelings onto your baby. You may think that your child is suffering because he needs you or that he is sad when you depart. And while these things may be true, your child will adjust—probably more quickly than you will. You may even worry that your child is adjusting too well to being in someone else's care. Don't worry—this does not mean that you are not needed. You may try to overcompensate for your absence by not setting limits with your child when you're at home. Many working parents feel that they do not get to see their child enough during the day, so they keep him up later at night. You may be more likely to respond to your child in the middle of the night, worried that your child needs you and will feel totally abandoned if you are not available at all hours of the night and are gone during the day.

Donna had a difficult time with the transition back to work. Donna worked for a large corporation and had to return to work when her baby, Megan, was six weeks old. Soon after Donna's return to work, Megan began to suffer from colic. For the next two months Megan screamed every day from 3:30 p.m. until midnight. The only time that Donna had good quality time with Megan was from 4:00 to 6:00 a.m., when Megan would awaken and Donna would nurse her. These were difficult times. It was stressful for Donna to be at work and away from Megan all day. Then, when she got home at 5:30, she would find a screaming baby, an exhausted babysitter, and a six-hour-long nighttime siege with a crying baby. During this time Megan slept much of the day and was awake much of the night. She reluctantly took a bottle during the day when she was with her babysitter, but she refused to take a bottle during the night when Donna was around. Even after the colic resolved, Megan continued to be a nighttime baby. She would sleep from 8:00 a.m. until 3:00 p.m., waking only for a four-ounce bottle around 11:30 a.m. When Donna came home, she would nurse Megan, who would then go back to sleep from 7:00 p.m. until 10:00 p.m. After that, Megan would wake up every two hours throughout the night to nurse and play. Donna felt guilty not being around during the day and believed that Megan was suffering because basically the only time that she would eat was when Donna was there to breast-feed her. At six months Megan seemed to be thriving, but Donna was exhausted.

The experience that Donna had with Megan is common. Returning to work often occurs before everyone is ready. The mother may not feel fully recovered physically and may not feel emotionally ready to be away from her newborn. The baby may not yet have a firmly established sleeping and feeding routine. And guilt often takes over. To help alleviate guilt, make sure that you feel comfortable with and confident about the person(s) caring for your baby. This will make the time that you are away easier. Then, once you have gotten adjusted to your return to work, step back and evaluate your life and your baby's life. Is everyone getting what he or she needs? Is there a better way to meet these needs? Is your baby waking during the night to eat because she truly needs the nutrition or because this has become a learned habit? Your baby needs a happy and functioning mother more than she needs to see you at 3:00 a.m. This may be a difficult transition period for you, but everyone has to be happy and functioning for a family to work.

Employees who work evening or night shifts may have even more difficulties with their baby's sleep. These individuals often have problems with their own sleep because they adjust to a day schedule on their days off. They also may not be able to get enough sleep because other demands are made on their time off during the day, such as child care. For those with changing shifts, their work schedule may wreak absolute havoc on their sleep. Their own sleep schedule may be so disorganized that it will inevitably affect their baby's schedule. Although there may not be much that you can do about your own daily schedule, try to keep your baby's schedule as consistent as possible. No matter whose care she is in, put her to bed at the same time every night and keep a tight schedule for her naps. This may take some work to accomplish, but it will be well worth it for your baby. She needs to keep a regular and consistent schedule in order to develop and grow up happy and content.

SEPARATION AND DIVORCE

The period surrounding separation and divorce can be a time of great upheaval for both parents and children. Children often do not understand what is going on. Many children blame themselves for Mommy's or Daddy's moving out, believing that they did something wrong to cause the separation or divorce. Young children often become much more clingy. If there is a great deal of arguing, children may become withdrawn or may tend to act out more. Although this is a difficult time for parents, much attention must be given to the children in this situation.

Sleep problems are likely to occur during and after the separation for a number of reasons. Your child's daily routine may be upset, and therefore she is less likely to have set naptimes and bedtimes. You may become more lenient with your child and less likely to set limits. Parents who are going through such upheaval may be more likely to allow and even want their child to share their bed. Also, when there are two separate homes, there may be two separate sets of rules regarding sleep and other matters concerning the child.

Don't worry: if you do all the wrong things in the beginning, it is understandable. But once things have calmed down, you must begin to deal with issues such as sleep problems. Remember, though, that prevention is the best solution to most problems. If you can prevent either the onset or the continuation of problems, that is best for you and your child.

If your child was already a good sleeper, stick to what you always did. Your child will feel much more secure if her routine stays the same. Try to retain your child's normal daily schedule. Keep naptimes the same. Put her to bed the same time every night. Have the same nightly routine. If the parent who was involved in the nighttime routine is no longer in the home, the other parent should try to do the same routine. If parts of the routine are not comfortable for that parent, then he or she should simply do what is comfortable and substitute something else for what would be uncomfortable. For example, if your wife always sang your baby a song at night and you can't sing, then come up with something that you can do, such as reading a book or telling a story.

Things can become difficult if your child sleeps at different times at each parent's home. For both your own and your child's sake, learn to communicate about parenting issues with the other parent. Parenting issues are not the ground on which to wage the battle concerning your marital problems. Your marriage may be over, but you will be joint parents for life. The best thing that you can do for your children is to maintain some semblance of peace about how to manage them. Try to set the same limits about sleep. Your child may have a difficult time sleeping at first, so try to have each parent maintain the same time for going to bed and a similar bedtime routine.

Be careful about giving in and letting your child stay up later or not have to sleep in his own bed. Good quality time with your child should occur at non–sleep times, not after bedtime. To help your baby sleep at both homes, make sure that your baby's favorite blanket and toy travel with her. Keep the beds similar as well: if she sleeps in a crib in one household, have her sleep in a crib in the other. If she sleeps in a bed, have the same at the other residence.

Should you let your child begin to sleep with you after a separation or divorce? If your child has always slept with you, then go ahead and continue. If not, you need to ask yourself why cosleeping is happening now. Is it for your sake or your child's? It is nice to have a warm body next to you in the middle of the night, but your child is not a substitute for your spouse. In addition, a sudden shift to cosleeping can be confusing for your child. This is especially true if your child is blaming herself in any way for the divorce. She may feel that she is replacing the parent who moved out. Psychologically, this is not good for your child. It will lead to ambivalent feelings about her relationship with both parents and her role in the family. Remember, she is the child and should remain the child in the relationship. For a more complete discussion of cosleeping, be sure to read Chapter 8.

If your child has always had sleep problems, this is not the time to decide to do something about them. Yes, sleep problems should be corrected, and your child needs to be taught to put herself to sleep and to sleep through the night. However, this is not the time. Wait until things have calmed down, some time after the separation. On the other hand, if the separation or divorce occurred a while ago, don't put off doing something about your child's sleep problems. Don't use the separation or divorce as an excuse to delay.

DEATH IN THE FAMILY

A death in the family, whether sudden or expected, is a tragic event. Your child will likely be experiencing grief, no matter what his age. Whether he is four months or three years old, your child will understand that something is wrong and will miss the person who died. If it is a relative or friend your child did not know well, he will still sense your grief and the atmosphere of crisis. If it is a grandparent or relative your child knows well, or worse yet, a parent, it is even more difficult. (Because this book is focused on sleep, only those pertinent issues will be discussed. However, be sure to get information on how to deal with your child regarding death and grief.)

People often explain death to young children as sleep. "Grandpa went to sleep and isn't going to ever wake up." This is not advisable. Children take things literally, at absolute face value. Your young child is going to believe that anyone who goes to sleep may not ever wake up again—and that includes you and your child. Your child may suddenly become terrified to go to sleep at night, afraid that he will die in his sleep. He may be afraid that you will die in your sleep. So whatever you do, don't explain death in terms of sleep.

After a death, the sleep issues that are likely to arise are similar to those discussed above for children experiencing their parents' separation or divorce. Many of these problems revolve around changes in routine. During the period after the death and throughout the funeral and mourning period, your child's schedule is apt to be different from the usual. Naptimes may be missed and late nights are likely. If the funeral is out of town, your child may have to adjust to sleeping in a hotel or at a relative's or friend's home. Even if the funeral takes place where you live, some families find it easier to have their children stay at others' homes. In such cases, try to bring along something comforting and familiar for your child, such as his favorite stuffed animal and his blanket and pillow. This sense of familiarity will help make the transition easier. If possible, try to maintain your child's usual naptimes and bedtime. If you will be unavailable to put her to sleep, have someone do it whom your child knows and feels comfortable with. If the death is of a parent—and especially if it is the parent who usually does the bedtime routine—try to mimic your child's usual routine as much as possible. Do things in the same order. If the child insists, "That's not the way Daddy did it," go along with your child's wishes. This is not the time to establish new ways of doing things. Expect your child to act up during this time, especially at bedtime. He is most likely not getting as much attention as usual, he may be overtired and cranky from missed sleep, and he may be reacting to the surrounding stress and tension. If possible, spend an extra few minutes cuddling; don't rush through the bedtime routine, and remain calm if he gets overly silly or cranky. If your child dawdles or becomes obstinate, take this as his way of reacting to the death rather than perceiving it as belligerence.

Another issue that may arise following a death is whether to allow your child to sleep with you. If this is your usual practice, don't insist on your child's sleeping alone all of a sudden. If your child normally sleeps in his own crib or bed, however, then you will need to consider the ramifications of this change in sleeping arrangements.

Another common sleep problem when a death occurs is for children older than age two to begin having nightmares about death and about the person who died. Your child may even dream about others dying. He may dream about dying himself or being lost. Nightmares of other bad things are also apt to occur. This is the time for lots of reassurance. For other suggestions on how to deal with nightmares, see Chapter 14.

Death is an issue that everyone has to deal with at some time. It can be especially difficult for young children because their understanding of death is limited. Expect this time to be difficult on everyone, and anticipate how you are going to deal with any sleep problems that arise.

Reminders ——————————————————————

- ✦ Even after your baby is sleeping through the night, antic-ipate obstacles to continued good sleep, such as vaca-tions and illness.
- ✦ Switching from a crib to a bed can be an easy transition for you and your toddler.
- ✦ Returning to work can disrupt everyone's schedule, as can the birth of a new baby.
- ✦ Changes in the family, including separation, divorce, or death, can disrupt sleep.

PART FOUR

Other Common Sleep Problems

CHAPTER 12

Snoring and Snorting: Sleep Apnea

"Doctor, you have to help me. Every night my son, Stevie, stops breathing. It lasts so long that I think he won't start breathing again. I have him sleep with me so that I can shake him to make him breathe whenever he stops. I have called our pediatrician because some nights he stops breathing for so long it scares me. But the doctor says he is perfectly fine."

WHAT IS SLEEP APNEA?

Sleep apnea, also known as obstructive sleep apnea, is a serious disorder in which there are pauses in breathing during sleep. Sleep apnea is generally thought of as a disorder that occurs in adults, but children often experience it. For some children, like Stevie, apnea is serious, and the parents, while aware of the problem, don't know where to turn for help. In many instances, however, the parents aren't even aware that their child has sleep apnea and do not seek medical help.

SYMPTOMS OF SLEEP APNEA IN CHILDREN

There are a number of symptoms to look for that are common in children with sleep apnea. Some children will have most of these symptoms, whereas others may have only one or two.

+ **Snoring**. Almost all children and adults who have sleep apnea snore. However, it is important to realize that not all children who snore have sleep apnea. Children with sleep apnea usually snore loudly, and most of the time (not just when they have a cold).
+ **Breathing pauses**. Breathing pauses are the hallmark of sleep apnea. Rather than breathing in an even and consistent manner, your child may stop breathing for a few moments and then start breathing again. If you observe this behavior, it is almost certain that your child has sleep apnea.
+ **Difficulty breathing while sleeping**. Rather than observing breathing pauses, you may notice that your child seems to have difficulty breathing while asleep. His breathing may not appear regular and even, or he may be a noisy breather.
+ **Mouth breathing**. Most children with obstructive sleep apnea breathe through their mouths at night—and often during the day as well.
+ **Coughing or choking**. If your child frequently starts coughing or choking in his sleep, this may be a sign of a breathing problem.
+ **Restless sleep**. Many children with sleep apnea are restless sleepers. Each time they have a breathing pause they will arouse and move.
+ **Sleeping in unusual positions**. Some children with sleep apnea sleep in an unusual position, for example, with

their head hanging over the side of the bed or with their head raised on several pillows or on stuffed animals. They do this unconsciously to try to keep their airway open to help them breathe while asleep.

✦ **Sweating.** Many children with sleep apnea sweat profusely while they sleep. The reasons for this are unclear, but it may be because the body has to work hard to breathe during sleep.

✦ **Nightmares or sleep terrors.** Children with sleep apnea may be more prone to these two sleep problems. The next chapter discusses both nightmares and sleep terrors.

✦ **Night wakings.** Frequent night wakings in infants and toddlers are usually related to sleep associations, as discussed in earlier chapters. However, some children's night wakings are caused by sleep apnea. If your child has other symptoms discussed in this chapter and awakens at night, it is worth considering whether or not your child has sleep apnea. Remember, though, that although his waking may be caused by the sleep apnea, he should be able to fall back to sleep on his own. If he does not, be sure also to consider a sleep association problem.

DAYTIME SYMPTOMS OFTEN ASSOCIATED WITH SLEEP APNEA IN CHILDREN

✦ **Appearing sleepy during the day.** Children with sleep apnea are not getting enough sleep because their nighttime sleep is interrupted so frequently. Thus, your child may be sleepy during the day. He may be difficult to get up in the morning and may fall asleep in school or at other unusual times (such as during meals). Younger children may nap longer or take more naps than others their age.

✦ **Appearing hyperactive during the day**. Many children who do not get enough sleep do not look and act sleepy. Instead, they become wired and hyperactive. This is common. Don't fool yourself by saying that your child is never tired because he is in constant motion. This may actually be a sign that he is overtired.

✦ **Daytime behavior problems**. Some children may have daytime behavior problems. For example, some children with sleep apnea are irritable, cranky, or easily frustrated. Others may have difficulty focusing their attention.

✦ **Behavior has changed significantly**. If your child's behavior has changed significantly during the day, such as appearing more cranky, irritable, or sleepy, and if he also has other symptoms that are discussed above, the problem may be associated with sleep apnea.

✦ **Falling asleep at inappropriate times or at times other than naptime**. Your child may not be getting enough sleep if he is falling asleep at inappropriate times. For example, does he always fall asleep while riding in the car, whether for a two-minute or twenty-minute drive? Does he fall asleep at mealtimes?

✦ **Health problems**. Many children with sleep apnea have a history of chronic problems with tonsils, adenoids, and/or ear infections.

✦ **Difficulty eating**. Some children with sleep apnea are noisy eaters, probably because they have difficulty breathing solely through their nose while chewing. Other children with sleep apnea are slow eaters, and some even have problems swallowing, especially if they have very large tonsils.

✦ **Slow growth**. Sleep apnea may cause growth impairment, as growth hormone gets released during sleep. Children with growth impairment are usually underweight and short for their age. If your child's growth is impaired because of sleep apnea, she may have a sudden growth spurt when the sleep apnea is treated and catch up to other children her age.

ADDITIONAL SYMPTOMS ASSOCIATED WITH SLEEP APNEA IN OLDER CHILDREN (AGES SIX AND UP)

+ **Bed-wetting.** Older children with sleep apnea often continue to wet their beds beyond when you would expect them to stay dry all night. If your older child is continuing to wet his bed, check to make sure that he doesn't have any of the symptoms listed above.
+ **Morning headache.** Some children with sleep apnea will complain of having a headache in the morning. The headache is caused by the decrease in oxygen to the brain during the night. This diminished oxygen is unlikely to be harmful, although it sounds scary. This symptom may also occur in infants and toddlers, although it is difficult to know whether they have a headache.
+ **Difficulty in school.** In older children the effects of sleep apnea may result in poor performance in school. These children may be labeled slow or lazy and may have difficulty focusing their attention on their schoolwork.

WILL SHE STOP BREATHING ALTOGETHER?

"Several times during the night my two-year-old seems to stop breathing. I am scared that she won't breathe again!"

Other than in cases of SIDS (discussed later in this chapter), your baby will always start breathing again. The body has its own internal mechanism to make sure that breathing continues. The pause in breathing during apnea triggers the body to awaken, which results in a return of muscle tone to the airway, and breathing resumes. These wakings are so brief that you and your child may not even be aware of them, but they disrupt normal, restorative sleep.

CAUSES OF SLEEP APNEA IN CHILDREN

The most common cause of obstructive sleep apnea in children is enlargement of the adenoids and tonsils. During sleep there is a considerable drop in muscle tone, which affects the airway and breathing. Many of these children have little difficulty breathing when awake; however, with decreased muscle tone during sleep, the airway becomes smaller, making the flow of air more difficult and the work of breathing harder. An analogy can be made to breathing through a small, flimsy straw with the straw occasionally collapsing and obstructing airflow. These obstructions result in frequent brief arousals from sleep. Many of the short pauses (lasting only a few to twenty seconds or so) cause a brief arousal that increases muscle tone, opens the airway, and allows the child to resume breathing. Although the actual number of minutes of arousal during the night may be small, the repeated, chronic, but brief disruptions in sleep can lead to significant daytime symptoms in children. A comparable image is being poked in the arm every few minutes throughout the night. The child is usually unaware of waking up, and the parent often describes the child as having very restless sleep but not necessarily waking up completely.

WHO IS AT RISK FOR SLEEP APNEA?

A number of factors put children at risk for sleep apnea. These include:

+ **Tonsils and adenoids.** As mentioned earlier, most children with sleep apnea have enlarged tonsils and/or adenoids. Once the muscles in the neck relax during sleep, the big tonsils or adenoids block the airway and impede breathing.

+ **Illness.** Children with frequent ear infections, sore throats, and tonsillitis are more likely to have sleep apnea. Allergies and asthma also can contribute to sleep apnea.

+ **Weight.** Sleep apnea is more common in children who are overweight, as the extra weight around their necks can make their airways smaller. Not all children with sleep apnea are overweight, however. Many children of normal weight have sleep apnea, and children with sleep apnea can even be underweight.

+ **Physical structure.** Other children who are at high risk for sleep apnea include those with abnormal bone structure in the jaw area. For instance, children who have a receding chin may have a smaller airway. Another potential cause may be a cleft palate, particularly if it has been repaired.

+ **Decreased muscle tone.** Children with decreased muscle tone, as a result of such conditions as cerebral palsy or muscular dystrophy, are at risk for sleep apnea.

+ **Down syndrome.** Children with Down syndrome are at risk for sleep apnea because they are often slightly overweight and because they often have an enlarged tongue that can block the airway during sleep. Studies have shown that almost half of all children with Down syndrome have sleep apnea.

SLEEP APNEA AND ADHD

There has recently been much focus on the relationship between sleep apnea and ADHD (attention deficit/hyperactivity disorder) in children. Studies have found that snoring is one and a half times more likely in children with ADHD. Another study indicated that up to 25 percent of children with ADHD may have some type of sleep-disordered breathing. These figures do not mean that all children with ADHD have sleep apnea, but it should definitely be considered. Not only has ADHD been focused on, but other behavioral and academic difficulties common with sleep apnea have been looked at in relationship to ADHD. For example, studies have found that 10–15 percent of children with academic problems have sleep apnea.

PREVALENCE OF SLEEP APNEA IN CHILDREN

Although it used to be considered rare, recent studies have shown that sleep apnea is more common in children than previously thought. Sleep apnea occurs in about 1–3 percent of all children. Sleep apnea can occur at any age but peaks between two and six years of age. There is no sex difference in the prevalence of sleep apnea; boys and girls are equally likely to have sleep apnea.

Snoring is much more common than sleep apnea. Occasional snoring occurs in about 20 percent of all children and nightly snoring in about 10 percent. Thus, just because your child snores does not mean that he has sleep apnea, but he should be evaluated.

FAMILY HISTORY

"My husband snores and so does our eleven-month-old baby. Is snoring inherited?"

Sleep apnea can run in families. Some children with sleep apnea have one or both parents with the same problem. Therefore, if you have been diagnosed with sleep apnea, it is a good idea to determine whether your child has any of the symptoms that were discussed above (for further information on sleep apnea in adults, see Chapter 16).

WHOM SHOULD YOU SEE FOR HELP?

Children with suspected sleep apnea should be seen by a sleep specialist. An extensive interview, a physical examination, and an overnight sleep study will likely be conducted. To find an accredited sleep disorders center near you, contact the American Academy of Sleep Medicine at (708)492–0930 or go to their Web site at www.aasmnet.org. Also, check with your physician about a sleep center in your area.

ASSESSMENT OF SLEEP APNEA IN CHILDREN

Jacob is five years old. His parents noticed that he always seemed to be sleepy during the day. At first they thought that Jacob just needed more sleep, but even with lots of sleep he still seemed sleepy.

He always fell asleep in the car, and his kindergarten teacher said that he fell asleep in school on a number of occasions, not just at naptime. Jacob's sleepiness was confusing to his parents, as Jacob was also a very active kid who had a hard time sitting still. His parents noted that he snored at night (it was a running joke in the family as to who snored louder—Jacob or his father), and he was a very restless sleeper. He breathed through his mouth both during the day and at night. Finally, concerned about Jacob's sleep, they mentioned the problem to their pediatrician. Their pediatrician referred them to a sleep disorders center.

After Jacob's parents made an appointment for the next week, they received a packet in the mail that included information about the center and a ten-page questionnaire to complete prior to the appointment about Jacob and his sleep. It included questions about Jacob's evening activities, such as television watching, bedtime, and bedtime routines; how long it took for Jacob to fall asleep; details of any unusual behaviors during the night, such as sleepwalking; the quality of his breathing at night; and any night wakings. There were also questions about what time Jacob woke up in the morning, how sleepy he appeared during the day, his daytime behavior, and whether he took naps. Jacob's parents also were asked to keep track of Jacob's sleep by keeping a sleep diary until the appointment. During the first appointment, the doctor asked every conceivable question about Jacob's sleep and even about their own sleep. Jacob was also given a brief physical examination that included checking his height and weight and looking in his ears and throat. The doctor found that Jacob had enlarged tonsils and thought that his symptoms indicated sleep apnea. To be sure, though, they wanted to perform a polysomnography (PSG) during an overnight sleep study at their sleep center.

Jacob's overnight study was scheduled for three weeks later. His parents were instructed to bring him to the sleep center at 6:30 p.m. Since Jacob liked to sleep in one of his father's T-shirts at home, Jacob's mother had to go out and get him pajamas that had a separate top and bottom to be worn during the study, as recommended by the doctor. They brought Jacob's favorite video, the teddy bear he slept with, and lots of juice and snacks. It was decided that Jacob's mother would stay with Jacob overnight because she could take the next day off from work.

Getting Jacob hooked up for the sleep study was relatively easy. At first he was a bit anxious, but the technicians at the sleep center explained to him that the electrodes that would be attached to his skin were not needles; they would not pierce his skin but, rather, would be glued or taped on. They helped Jacob get over being scared by first putting some electrodes on his mother and then having Jacob put them on his bear. They also let him watch his video while they got him ready. He was finally hooked up and it was bedtime. Jacob had a hard time settling down at first, going to sleep in a strange bed with a bunch of wires attached, but with some reassurance from his mother he calmed down and went to sleep. During the night, the monitors kept track of Jacob's oxygen levels, how much air was going in and out of his nose and mouth (oral and nasal airflow), respiration, arm and leg muscle activity, and his brain waves by way of an electroencephalograph. The next morning when Jacob woke up, all the electrodes were removed, and his mother took him to school.

Jacob and his parents returned two weeks later for a follow-up appointment and were told that Jacob definitely had sleep apnea. They were referred to an ear, nose, and throat specialist. Eventually, Jacob had his tonsils and adenoids removed. His snoring and restless sleep resolved, as did his daytime sleepiness, and he appeared calmer and better able to focus during the day. Shortly after this, his father also made an appointment with a sleep center to be evaluated because of his snoring and feeling sleepy during the day.

As with Jacob, a thorough evaluation at a sleep disorders center typically involves: (1) obtaining a complete history of your child's sleep, (2) the keeping of a sleep diary for one to two weeks, (3) a physical examination, and (4) an overnight sleep study if an underlying physical problem is suspected. Following the collection of all of this information, a diagnosis and a treatment plan are made. The sleep disorders center staff will also send the findings to your pediatrician.

TREATMENT FOR CHILDHOOD SLEEP APNEA

For most children with sleep apnea, removal of the enlarged tonsils and adenoids is the first treatment. An ear, nose, and throat specialist will evaluate whether your child should have a tonsillectomy and/or adenoidectomy. Any doctor can see the tonsils, but special equipment is needed to see the adenoids. Once the tonsils and/or adenoids are removed, the airway will not be blocked, and breathing during sleep can occur normally. The surgery is usually done on an outpatient basis, meaning that your child will go to the hospital in the morning for surgery and be released that afternoon. Some children with moderate to severe sleep apnea, though, may be kept overnight to be sure that any postsurgery swelling does not make the child's apnea worse. Once the swelling has dissipated, the apnea usually disappears. There are few risks involved in this type of surgery, but it is always important to ask your doctor about any possible complications.

If other physical problems are causing obstruction, other procedures may be recommended. For example, if your child has nasal polyps or any other growths in his nose or throat, these will need to be removed. When the doctor is evaluating for a tonsillectomy and/or adenoidectomy, a complete inspection for these types of growths will be done at the same time. Sometimes a child will need correction of a deviated nasal septum, usually the result of a broken nose. In severe cases, correction of malformations of the jaw or upper palate may be necessary.

If the cause of your child's sleep apnea is related to asthma or allergies, these need to be brought under control. A pulmonologist or allergy specialist should be seen for these types of problems. For some children, weight loss may be beneficial in eliminating sleep apnea, but consult your pediatrician before starting any weight-loss program for your child.

Another effective treatment that is commonly prescribed for adults with sleep apnea is continuous positive airway pressure (CPAP), and this treatment is now becoming more common for children. In this highly effective therapy, a mask is worn over the nose during sleep, and pressure from an air compressor forces air through nasal passages and into the airway. This air pressure keeps the airway open and allows the child to breathe normally during sleep without the disturbing arousals.

SUDDEN INFANT DEATH SYNDROME (SIDS)

Any discussion of infant sleep is not complete without a discussion of sudden infant death syndrome (SIDS), a tragedy that occurs most often while a baby is sleeping. It is not likely to happen to your baby, but it is a possibility that you should take into account and do what you can to prevent.

After two years of trying, Lisa finally got pregnant, and she and John were happy to welcome Caitlin, a seven-pound two-ounce baby girl. Although the first few weeks were difficult for John and Lisa, mostly because of sleep deprivation, Caitlin was "perfect." She was healthy and gaining weight. Everyone said that she was adorable, and her pediatrician proclaimed her healthy and normal. She started smiling and holding her head up. She began sleeping through the night at nine weeks. John and Lisa were ecstatic about finally becoming parents. On a Tuesday night when Caitlin was thirteen weeks old,

Lisa put Caitlin to bed at 8:30 p.m. All was quiet throughout the night, as it usually was. By 8:00 a.m. Caitlin was still not awake, which was unusual. When Lisa went to check on her, she found that Caitlin was not breathing and was lifeless. The paramedics came but said there was nothing they could do. The police were called, and an autopsy was done. Nothing was found to have caused Caitlin's death. The final conclusion was sudden infant death syndrome, otherwise known as SIDS.

Unfortunately, babies do die in their sleep. Sudden infant death syndrome, also referred to as crib death or cot death, is the leading cause of death in infants between the ages of one month and one year. In the United States, about twenty-five hundred babies die each year from SIDS, a decrease of almost 50 percent compared to the 1980s. The definition of SIDS, according to the National Institutes of Health, is "the sudden death of an infant under one year of age, which remains unexplained after a complete postmortem examination, including an investigation of the death scene and a review of the case history." Thus, there is no clear cause of death.

Most babies who die of SIDS are between the ages of two and four months. Almost 90 percent of babies who die of SIDS are under six months of age. SIDS occurs slightly more often in boys than girls. Although it can happen at any time of the year, SIDS occurs most often in the fall and winter. SIDS rates are also highest among African Americans and American Indians, and lowest among Asians and Hispanics.

SIDS is not caused by child abuse. It is also not caused by vomiting or choking, or by minor illnesses, such as colds or infections. It is not contagious and it is not caused by immunizations for diseases, such as diphtheria or tetanus.

What Babies Are at Risk for SIDS?

It is impossible to identify exactly which babies are at risk for SIDS. We do know, however, about a number of trends regarding SIDS. For instance, the three most well-identified factors that place a baby at risk for SIDS are sleep position (stomach or side sleeping), exposure to smoke, and becoming overheated while sleeping. In addition, babies born to younger mothers are more at risk for SIDS, as are those with a sibling close in age. Twins and triplets are more at risk, as are babies who had a low birth weight. Brothers and sisters of SIDS victims are also more likely to suffer from SIDS, especially if there was more than one SIDS victim in the family. Maternal health can also place a baby at risk. Not only are mothers who smoke more likely to have a baby who dies of SIDS, but those who use alcohol or illegal drugs during pregnancy, have a history of sexually transmitted disease or urinary tract infections, are anemic, or receive poor prenatal care also place their babies at higher risk.

Although breast-feeding is clearly beneficial, studies do not indicate a clear link between breast-feeding and reduced risk of SIDS. Interestingly, some studies have found lower rates of SIDS in babies who use pacifiers.

Surprisingly, most babies who are victims of SIDS were considered healthy prior to their death and were well developed and nourished. Most babies were also full-term, meaning that they were not born substantially early. Many do not even have any of the risk factors mentioned here.

SIDS and Child Care Settings

Recent research indicates that 20 percent of SIDS deaths occur in child care settings. One possible reason is that there is not as much awareness of the risk of certain practices, such as smoke exposure, soft bedding, and unsafe sleeping environments. In addition, babies may be more likely to be placed on their stomach or side to sleep. Not only are these sleep positions unsafe, but babies who are unaccustomed to sleeping in these positions are even more at risk. Thus, be sure to speak to your child care provider about safe sleeping practices and insist that your baby be placed on his or her back at all sleep times, including naps.

What Causes SIDS?

No one really knows what causes SIDS, and in fact it is likely that there are many reasons why babies die from SIDS. Current theory is that certain babies are vulnerable to external stressors, likely a result of subtle abnormalities in the brain. These defects appear to be related to the part of the nervous system that controls breathing and heart rate. Much remains to be learned about the causes of SIDS, and thus prevention, of this tragic event.

What Can Be Done to Prevent SIDS?

Unfortunately, we don't know of a way to prevent SIDS completely. The following recommendations, however, will help reduce your baby's risk of being a victim of SIDS.

SLEEP POSITION. First, have your young infant sleep on his back. Babies who sleep on their stomach are more susceptible to SIDS. In the past, pediatricians recommended that babies sleep on their stomach or side because there were concerns that babies might choke if they vomited while asleep on their back. Research indicates that this is unlikely. However, studies have found a significant decrease in SIDS in babies who sleep on their back; in fact, getting infants to sleep on their back is the basis of "Back to Sleep," a national campaign to inform parents that this is the preferred sleep position for babies. This campaign has been highly successful and has reduced the incidence of SIDS by almost 50 percent. Not only has this campaign been launched in the United States, but it has been instituted worldwide with great success.

At some point your baby may decide that he wants to sleep on his stomach and will keep rolling into this position throughout the night. Most babies who are able to roll over onto their stomach are past the high-risk SIDS period. Speak with your pediatrician if this happens, to be sure that your baby is not at risk for SIDS. With your pediatrician's approval your baby can sleep this way.

STOP SMOKING AROUND THE BABY. Studies have shown that mothers who smoke throughout pregnancy and following the birth of their baby triple the risk of their baby's dying from SIDS. Surprisingly, women who quit smoking during pregnancy but return to smoking once the baby is born have babies who are twice as at risk for SIDS. So smoking should not take place near your baby.

USE FIRM BEDDING. Babies should sleep on a firm, flat mattress. Babies should not sleep on beanbag cushions, sheepskins, foam pads, quilts, pillows, or any other soft item. These soft items can be dangerous because your baby can easily smother. Also avoid having your baby sleep on a waterbed, sofa, or any other soft surface.

AVOID OVERHEATING YOUR BABY. SIDS has been associated with babies who are overheated by too much clothing, too many blankets, or too warm a room. This is especially true for a baby with a cold or infection. You can tell if your baby is overheated by whether she is sweating, has damp hair or a heat rash, or is breathing rapidly. Dress your baby in as much or as little clothing as you are wearing. It is also best to dress your baby in nighttime clothing such that no other blankets or other coverings are necessary, such as a footed blanket sleeper during the winter months. Finally, keep bedrooms at a consistent 68 to 70 degrees Fahrenheit.

HOME APNEA MONITORING. Some parents utilize home monitors, which alert them if their baby stops breathing or if there is a problem with the baby's heart rate. These monitors are helpful, although they are not guaranteed to avert all SIDS occurrences. Typically, the babies who are most likely to be placed on home monitors include those who have had a past life-threatening event, premature babies with apnea, the twin of a SIDS victim, babies born to families in which there have been two or more prior SIDS victims, and infants with existing heart or breathing problems. Home monitoring is not recommended for normal infants and healthy preterm infants.

The Impact of SIDS

SIDS occurs unexpectedly and suddenly. Babies are not supposed to die. The first few months after a baby is born is a time of joy and bonding with the new baby, and the unexpected death of a baby is especially traumatic. The first reactions are usually numbness and bewilderment. As one parent simply stated, "This wasn't supposed to happen." Since there is no one to blame for the death, parents often blame themselves, thinking, "If only I had checked on him." The parents often perceive themselves as failures and question why they hadn't noticed any problems or done anything to protect their baby. And, as if to compound the pain, some SIDS deaths involve legal investigations into the baby's death, sometimes with fingers being pointed at the parents.

After the initial shock, many parents become severely depressed. They may have difficulties concentrating and sleeping. They may become tired and irritable. They may have difficulty functioning, at home and at work. If there are other children in the family, parents may become overprotective, never letting them out of their sight.

Another common occurrence after the death of a child to SIDS is moving to a new home. Many couples can't live with any remembrances of their child and try to change as many aspects of their life as they can, in an attempt to escape the painful memories. Fears about future pregnancies and having another baby are also extremely common.

The death of a baby to SIDS will affect other children in the family as well. The death will be just as traumatic for them. Some children may feel that it is their fault, especially if they felt any resentment toward the new baby who was the center of attention. They may worry that they will die in their sleep. Most will be confused about the death and unable to understand what happened. Some children will become withdrawn. The other children in the family are going to need support. They will need to have the death explained to them in a way that is appropriate for their age. They will need to understand that it is normal and important to grieve and feel sad. Parents will need to help their children deal with their own feelings.

If your baby is a victim of SIDS, get support. Most parents whose babies die of SIDS feel guilty, but you must remember that it is not your fault and there was nothing that you could have done to prevent it. Be sure to contact a local chapter of the SIDS Alliance. Phone numbers and addresses for such organizations can be found in Appendix B, "Resources for Parents."

If you know someone who has lost a child to SIDS, you should realize that the parents need support. This does not mean that you need to make them feel better. Pain and grieving, which may continue for months and years after the death of the child, are important aspects of their recovery. Parents of SIDS victims often want to talk about the baby, and they don't mind when others talk about their child. Don't be reluctant to talk about the baby. This will not upset the parents. The baby did exist, and parents often enjoy talking about him and appreciate someone listening to their stories. The parents may also appreciate tangible reminders of their baby, so feel free to give or make something, such as a framed picture of the baby. Give a donation in memory of the baby or plant a tree in his honor. All of these gestures will be appreciated.

Being a friend and listening, though, are probably the best things you can do.

Reminders

+ Sleep apnea is a serious disorder in which there are pauses in breathing during sleep.
+ Common nighttime symptoms of sleep apnea in children are snoring, breathing pauses, mouth breathing, and difficulty breathing while asleep.
+ Common daytime symptoms of sleep apnea include appearing sleepy, hyperactivity, and falling asleep at inappropriate times.
+ Enlarged tonsils or adenoids are the predominant cause of sleep apnea in children.
+ A diagnosis of sleep apnea should be made at a sleep disorders center.
+ Sudden infant death syndrome (SIDS) is the leading cause of death in infants between the ages of one month and one year. There are things that you can do to help prevent SIDS, especially having your baby sleep on his or her back.

CHAPTER 13

Babies Who Go Bump in the Night: Parasomnias

"Every night around 10:30 Billy bolts out of bed and starts scream-ing uncontrollably. I often find him running around his room looking frantic. I try to hold him, but he just pushes me away. I don't under-stand what is happening. He looks terrified, and it frightens me."

Unusual behaviors that occur during sleep are called parasomnias. Billy's nighttime behavior is known as a sleep terror or night terror. Parasomnias are common in babies and toddlers. In time, most chil-dren grow out of these unusual sleep disturbances. For parents, how-ever, watching their toddler have a sleep terror can be a very frightening experience.

PARASOMNIAS

The term "parasomnia" refers to a wide variety of behaviors that oc-cur during sleep. The most common type of parasomnia is the "disor-der of partial arousal," which includes confusional arousals, sleepwalking, and sleep terrors. These three sleep problems are all ba-sically the same thing but exist on a continuum from mild to severe. Essentially, they arise when the child is in a mixed state, being both asleep and awake, generally coming from the deepest stage of non-dreaming sleep (stages three and four of non-REM sleep). The child is awake enough to act out complex behaviors, but asleep enough not to be aware of or remember them. These events are usually infrequent and mild. However, they may occur often enough or be sufficiently severe or bothersome to require medical attention.

Confusional Arousals

Confusional arousals usually begin with crying and thrashing around in the crib or bed. Your child will appear awake and may look confused or upset. She may moan or cry out, but if you try to comfort her, she may resist you and not allow you to console her. You will realize that she is half asleep, and she will be difficult to awaken. These episodes may last up to half an hour. They usually end with a child calming down and returning to a deep sleep. Sometimes a child will awaken briefly from a confusional arousal, only to return to sleep quickly.

Most infants and toddlers have had at least one confusional arousal. It may have happened to your child without your even realizing it. Often a child who "wakes up" after being asleep for only an hour or so is having one of these events. It may just seem to you that your child seemed to wake up, fuss for a while, and then fell back to sleep. As stated before, most children have confusional arousals. They are extremely common and primarily occur in children under the age of three.

Sleepwalking

Sleepwalking is often seen in older children, peaking in children between the ages of four and eight. Up to half of all children have at least one episode of sleepwalking, with 3–4 percent sleepwalking frequently. Some children will simply get out of bed and walk around the room, whereas other children may sleepwalk for a long period and may go to another part of the house or even outside to the yard or garage. The sleepwalker may return to bed or awaken in the morning in a different part of the house, such as in a closet or someone else's room. Sleepwalkers can carry on conversations, which are difficult to understand and make little or no sense. Children who are sleepwalking are capable of acting out complicated behaviors, such as getting a snack, but usually the activities make little sense. It is quite common for children, especially boys, to urinate in closets or other strange places while sleepwalking. When your child sleepwalks, his eyes will be open, but they may appear "glassy."

Sleep Terrors

Sleep terrors, or night terrors as they are often called, are the most extreme and dramatic form of partial-arousal disorders. They are also the most distressing to witness. Sleep terrors usually begin with a bloodcurdling scream or shout. During one of these events your child may look as though she is experiencing extreme terror. Her pupils may be dilated, she will breathe rapidly, her heart will be racing, and she may be sweating. Overall, she will look extremely agitated. During a sleep terror a child may bolt out of bed and run around the room or even out of the house. During a very frenzied event, children may hurt themselves or someone trying to calm them. As disturbing and frightening as these events appear to the observer, children having them are totally unaware of what they are doing and do not remember the incident in the morning. In fact, sleep terrors are much worse to watch than to experience. For the child, a sleep terror is less traumatic than a typical nightmare or bad dream. An easy way to distinguish between sleep terrors and nightmares is to determine who is more upset the next morning. If your child is more upset, then it was a nightmare. If you are more upset, then it was a sleep terror.

About 3 percent of children have sleep terrors, with most sleep terrors occurring when the child is between five and seven years, although younger children can also have them.

While the term "parasomnia" refers to a wide range of sleep disorders, for the rest of this chapter, "parasomnia" will refer to these three disorders of partial arousal: confusional arousals, sleepwalking, and sleep terrors.

CRUCIAL FEATURES

Confusional arousals, sleepwalking, and sleep terrors all have a number of characteristics in common that distinguish them from other sleep disorders. Once you know about these features, these disorders are relatively easy to identify.

+ **Time of night**. Parasomnias usually occur within one to two hours of falling asleep. They also occur like clockwork. That is, you may be able to predict almost to the minute what time your child is going to have one. Don's son, Matthew, goes to bed every night at 8:30 and falls asleep by 9:00. At 10:15, Matthew starts screaming. This happens at least twice a week. If Don hasn't heard Matthew by 10:30, he knows that there will be no sleep terror that night. Note, though, that some children sleepwalk or have a sleep terror later in the night, or even during a nap.
+ **Amnesia**. Another feature of parasomnias is that your child will have no memory of these events. In the morning, to them, it will be as if it had never happened. Some children, if they have them often enough, may have

some fuzzy recollection of being up but no more than that.

✦ **Avoid comfort**. Children who are upset usually cling to their parents. Children having a parasomnia do not. They may not appear to even notice you. They are likely to scream more if you pick them up or try to hold them. They may get more upset if you talk to them and try to calm them down. Just leave them alone. Watch them, but don't interfere.

WHAT PARASOMNIAS ARE AND ARE NOT

We don't know what exactly parasomnias are, but we do know some things about them. All parasomnias occur during non-REM sleep (which was discussed in Chapter 2). They occur during transitions from one sleep stage to another. They usually occur coming out of stage three or four sleep, what is referred to as deep sleep. During a parasomnia a child is basically stuck halfway between being asleep and awake. He is not fully asleep or fully awake.

Some children sleepwalk or have a sleep terror every night. For other children, it will wax and wane, with good weeks and bad weeks. Every child is different. Some children may have only one episode in their lifetime.

We also know that parasomnias are *not* any of the following:

✦ **Not a nightmare**. Sleep terrors are not nightmares. Your child is not dreaming during these events, although it may look it. Nightmares occur during REM sleep. Most of REM sleep occurs at the end of the sleep period, usually early in the morning. This means that nightmares are also more likely during the second half of the night. One of the defining characteristics of REM sleep is that you are basically paralyzed. Your eyes move, your heart pumps, and you are able to breathe, but you are not able to move. So you cannot yell, cannot sit up in bed, and definitely cannot walk. Sleepwalking, confusional arousals, and sleep terrors occur in non-REM sleep, when you are not dreaming and are not paralyzed.

✦ **Not a psychological problem**. Many parents become worried that sleep terrors and sleepwalking indicate that their child has a serious psychological problem. The child looks terrified and frightened. It may appear that he is acting out some concern or problem that occurred during daytime hours, but this is not so. Many studies have been done, and the consensus is that parasomnias are not related to psychological problems. The child does not have problems with anxiety and is not depressed, and he certainly is not psychotic or having hallucinations. He is simply stuck halfway between awake and asleep.

✦ **Not possessed**. Some parents say that their child looks possessed or is speaking "in tongues." Rita commented that Mark sounded as if he were speaking a language from another planet. This isn't true. Your child just looks and acts strange during a sleep terror.

DISTINGUISHING PARASOMNIAS FROM OTHER PROBLEMS

✦ **Nightmares**. It is very easy to distinguish parasomnias from nightmares if you know what to look for. The table on the next page compares parasomnias with nightmares on several key components.

✦ **Seizures**. Parasomnias can also be confused with seizures that occur during sleep. It is very unlikely that your child is having a seizure, because seizures are quite rare, but you should be aware of what to look for. Seizures can occur at

	Parasomnias	Nightmares
Time of night	First third of night	Mid to last third
Behavior	Variable	Very little motor
Level of consciousness	Unarousable or very confused if awakened	Fully awake
Memory of event	Amnesia	Vivid recall
Family history	Yes	No
Potential for injury	High	Low
Frequency	Common	Very common
Stage of sleep	Deep non-REM	REM
Daytime sleepiness	Little or none	None

any time of the night but often happen shortly after a child falls asleep. The behavior is repetitive and stereotypic, meaning that your child will move the same way over and over. You will not be able to arouse your child, and your child will not recall the event in the morning, similar to parasomnias. If your child is having seizures during sleep, he may also be sleepy during the day. Again, seizures in sleep are very rare compared to common parasomnias and nightmares. If you have any concern that your child may be having seizures, contact your child's doctor.

CAUSES

Just as we don't know exactly what parasomnias are, we also don't know what exactly causes them. We do know that they run in families. If a child has them, it is likely that one of his parents had them, although maybe not as severely. In some families every one of the children has them to some degree. They also appear to be a developmental phenomenon, with children most likely to have them at certain ages.

There are certain factors that cause these sleep disorders to be worse or more likely to occur.

SLEEP DEPRIVATION. Not getting enough sleep is the number one reason that a child has a sleep terror or walks in his sleep. If your child doesn't get enough sleep on Wednesday night, he is more likely to have a sleep terror on Thursday night. This is because confusional arousals, sleepwalking, and sleep terrors occur during deep sleep. When deprived of sleep, the body demands more deep sleep and gets more than usual on a normal night. So the more deep sleep your child gets, the more likely it is that he will have an episode.

MEDICATIONS. Some medications can cause parasomnias. Lithium, Prolixin, and desipramine can induce or exacerbate parasomnias. Chloral hydrate, which is given to some children to help them sleep, can lead to a parasomnia. Linda was having problems getting her two-year-old daughter to sleep through the night. Her doctor prescribed chloral hydrate. That night Linda found her daughter sleepwalking.

FEVERS OR ILLNESS. A high fever or being sick can cause confusional arousals and sleep terrors. The higher the fever, the more likely an event will occur. For some children, this is the only time that they will ever have parasomnias. If you have never observed one in your child before, it can be very scary, especially when your child is sick.

STRANGE PLACES. Sleeping at Grandma's house, a friend's house, or any new place can lead to a sleep terror or sleepwalking.

NOISE. An event can be triggered by noises, such as sirens and even the creaking of the door when a parent goes to check on a child during the night.

STRESSFUL TIMES. Parasomnias often occur during periods of stress. It is not the stress itself that causes the sleep problems but the sleep deprivation that often goes along with it. If you are moving or going through a divorce, or if there has been a death in the family, your child may not be getting to bed as early as you would like and may not be getting enough sleep. If your child is worrying before falling asleep, he may not be getting the sleep he needs. Whenever this happens, unusual sleep behaviors are more likely to occur.

OTHER SLEEP DISORDERS. Some children's parasomnias are made worse by another, underlying sleep disrupter. For example, if your child has sleep apnea, it may be causing her to wake more frequently, resulting in more sleep transitions and making her more sleep deprived. Both factors may trigger a sleep terror. One recent study found that a significant percentage of older children with sleep terrors also had sleep apnea. When the sleep apnea was treated, the sleep terrors resolved. The same is true if your child wakes frequently at night for other reasons, such as needing to be rocked back to sleep. Once the behavioral problem is resolved, often the sleep terrors go away. Therefore, it is important to evaluate whether a child having sleep terrors may be having other sleep problems.

GENETICS. Sleep terrors and sleepwalking often run in families. Studies find that 80–90 percent of children who have sleep terrors have a close family member who has or had similar episodes. Often a child with parasomnias has a parent who either walked in his sleep or had sleep terrors as a child. At the very least, the parent talked in his or her sleep or continues to do so (sleep talking is in the same family as these other disorders).

KEEP YOUR CHILD SAFE

Heather, age four, would often sleepwalk during the night. She would usually walk out of her room, turn left, and turn left again into the bathroom. One night, while staying at her grandmother's house, she began sleepwalking as usual. She walked out of the room and turned left. She then turned left again, expecting to walk into the bathroom. Unfortunately, in her grandmother's house there was a stairway leading downstairs. Heather fell down the stairs and broke her right arm.

———

Heather's story is typical. People can easily get injured sleepwalking when sleeping in an unfamiliar place, be it at a grandparent's house or at a friend's place. If your child has sleep terrors or is a known sleepwalker, be sure to use safety precautions both at home and wherever she sleeps.

The most common injuries occur when a sleepwalking child falls out of a second-story or higher window or walks outside. Surprisingly, although your child is asleep, he can still see. This is why, at home, he doesn't usually bump into furniture and is unlikely to fall down the stairs. In the dark or in a strange place, however, accidents can happen. And even for children who sleepwalk regularly without incident, it is possible for their sleepwalking patterns to suddenly change. Children have been found at a neighbor's house, down the street, and in driveways. Often they walk out of their room, go somewhere, lie down, and fall back to sleep, waking in the morning unsure of where they are.

The most important thing you can do is make sure that your child is safe. Just because your child has sleep terrors but has never sleepwalked in the past doesn't mean that he won't begin next week. It is better to be safe than sorry, especially if your child has ever had a parasomnia event. Here are some things you can do to make sure that your child is safe.

GATES. Put up gates at the door of your child's bedroom and at the top of stairs. For younger children, the gates will stop them from leaving their room or going downstairs. For older children, the gate may not stop them, but perhaps it will slow them down enough for someone to hear them.

ALARMS. An alarm can be very helpful in making sure that your child doesn't leave the house. An alarm is not intended to wake your child but to wake you. Any type of alarm will do, from burglar alarms to a simple and more economical option. For instance, hang a bell or other jangling item from a string in your child's doorway so that when the door opens, it will make noise. The sound doesn't have to wake your child, but it should be loud enough to wake you. There are also inexpensive burglar alarms available that hang on doorknobs. If the doorknob is touched or turned, a loud alarm goes off. There are fancy electric eye systems that you can install in your child's room, even over his bed, that will be triggered when your child gets up and starts moving about. A word of caution, though: if you are relying on an in-home alarm system, especially one that has motion sensors, be careful that the police don't get called simply because your child is sleepwalking.

LOCK WINDOWS. Ensure that windows, especially second-story or higher, do not open enough that your child can jump or fall out of them. There are devices available that prevent windows from opening more than a few inches.

REARRANGE FURNITURE. Rearrange the furniture in your child's room so that he won't bump into anything in the dark and get hurt. A low table in the middle of the room may be perfect for drawing on during the day but can be dangerous if your child is sleepwalking in the middle of the night.

REMOVE THINGS THAT ARE IN THE WAY. If your child walks in his sleep, clear away anything that he can step on or trip over during the night. Don't leave piles of blocks lying on the floor near the bedroom door, and be sure to pick up scattered toys.

SLEEPING ON THE FIRST FLOOR. If your child is in real danger of going out a second-story or higher window, consider having your child sleep on the first floor. If you live in a fifth-floor apartment, obviously you can't do this. But in other cases, this may be possible.

HOW TO DEAL WITH PARASOMNIAS

Following are suggestions of things you can do to deal with your child's parasomnias.

DON'T WAKE YOUR CHILD. Waking your child will not harm your child—that is an old wives' tale—but it will prolong the event.

GUIDE YOUR CHILD BACK TO BED. Your child is asleep during these events, although he may not look it. He will eventually, and sometimes abruptly, return to normal sleep. To encourage this, guide your child gently back to bed. If he resists, let him be.

TRY NOT TO INTERFERE TOO MUCH. The normal response of parents is to try to comfort their child during a parasomnia episode. Try to resist doing this. Most children will just get more agitated, especially if you try to hold a child who already appears upset. If your child is about to come to harm, though, be sure to keep him safe even if he fights you.

INCREASE AMOUNT OF SLEEP. Try to increase the length of time that your child is asleep in order to avoid sleep deprivation. Parasomnias are much more likely to happen when your child is sleep deprived. This is because confusional arousals, sleepwalking, and sleep terrors all occur during transitions from deep sleep. If your child is not getting enough sleep, he will have more deep sleep and will be more likely to have a parasomnia. So increase naptime and move bedtime earlier.

MAINTAIN A REGULAR SLEEP SCHEDULE. Parasomnias are more likely to happen on nights that your child goes to sleep at a different time from his usual bedtime. So stick with a schedule of going to bed and waking up at the same time every day.

DON'T DISCUSS THE EVENT THE NEXT DAY. The morning after an event, don't discuss the problem with your child. Discussing the event is likely to worry him. This can lead to your child's becoming anxious about going to sleep, because he is scared about what he may do. If he is anxious, he is less likely to fall asleep at night and then may become sleep deprived. This, unfortunately, can lead to even more events. In addition, discussing parasomnias may lead older brothers and sisters to tease a younger child about how "weird" he was last night.

ALLAY YOUR CHILD'S FEARS. Although this book is geared toward infants and toddlers, you may have an older child who has parasomnias. For an older child, it may be helpful to discuss how common these behaviors are and to allay your child's fears or concerns that he is different or that something is wrong with him. Many older children with parasomnias become worried that they are crazy. Such a discussion should occur as part of everyday conversation. It is still recommended, even with older children, that you not discuss whether such an event occurred the previous night. Again, it can make a child self-conscious and lead to avoidance of sleep.

TREATMENT OPTIONS

In most cases parasomnias require no treatment other than the suggestions above. After all, these events rarely indicate any serious underlying medical or psychiatric problem. Furthermore, the number of events tends to decrease as children get older; most children do not have them after puberty.

In severe cases, when parasomnias are extremely frequent or involve injury, violence, or disruption of others' sleep, treatment may be necessary. This treatment may include medical intervention with prescription drugs. No matter what treatment you choose—including doing nothing—make sure that your child is always safe and can't hurt himself.

Medications

Doctors usually try to avoid giving drugs to a child who has para-somnias. However, in certain instances, when the sleep terrors are extreme or the child is in danger of hurting himself or someone else, medication may be recommended.

Adolfo is five years old and has been having sleep terrors almost every night for the past eighteen months. They have gotten worse over time. Most nights he screams so loudly that he is hoarse the next day. His sleep terrors have also gotten violent. The week before he was evaluated at a sleep disorders center, he tried to throw a television set at his two-year-old sister. Now his sister is terrified of him. His mother hasn't slept in weeks because she is worried that some-one will get hurt. Adolfo has become so anxious about going to sleep at night that it now takes him hours to fall asleep, and this has made his sleep terrors even worse.

In a case like Adolfo's, medication is warranted. The most common types of medications given are benzodiazepines, such as Restoril or Klonopin. These drugs have a sedative effect and are often prescribed for anxiety. For parasomnias, though, they are prescribed not because of their effect on anxiety but because they are sedating and they may suppress deep sleep—which is when sleep terrors are most likely to occur. These drugs will also help your child fall asleep, an asset if your child is scared to go to sleep. Usually a very short-acting medication is prescribed because all that is needed is to cover the first few hours when sleep terrors occur. You also don't want a medication that stays in the system any longer than a few hours, because you don't want your child to be groggy and feeling sluggish the next day.

Reminders ────────────────────────────────

- ✦ Parasomnias are unusual behaviors that occur at night.
- ✦ Confusional arousals, sleepwalking, and sleep terrors are three parasomnias that children often experience.
- ✦ Parasomnias are the result of your child's being awake and asleep at the same time. They do not indicate any type of psychological problem.
- ✦ Many things can bring on a parasomnia, including sleep deprivation, certain medications, and fevers or illness.
- ✦ Make sure that you keep your child safe.
- ✦ There are ways to deal with parasomnias, including not waking your child and avoiding sleep deprivation.
- ✦ Other treatments for parasomnias are available, including medication.

CHAPTER 14

Mumbling and Grumbling: More Common Sleep Problems

"Benjamin is often scared at bedtime, and he won't stay in his room alone because of the monsters under his bed."

"Robert is only eight months old. Could he actually be having nightmares?"

"All night long I hear this incredible banging from my daughter Tiffany's room."

Many parents are concerned about bedtime fears, nightmares, head banging, or even teeth grinding. Unfortunately, future parents very seldom hear about these behaviors, and few, if any, parenting books discuss them.

BEDTIME FEARS

Bedtime fears are the most common fears experienced by young children. Situations in which they are alone and it is dark are prime times for children to be afraid. Bedtime fears typically involve being scared of the dark. This is part of normal development. Fear of the dark begins to develop as children start to realize that they can get hurt or be harmed. Once children understand this concept, it will take some time for them to comprehend what is likely to harm them versus what is not. It is important for children to learn how to cope with bedtime fears and recognize that they are not in danger. This is in contrast to a situation in which a child is not likely to be afraid but could possibly be in danger. Think of all the times when your parents told you never to accept candy from strangers or accept a ride from someone you didn't know. These situations seem safe to children because most adults with whom they have had contact are considered safe and have always been nice to them. Part of being a parent is helping your child to develop realistic fears and distinguish them from unrealistic fears. This process may take a while. Thus, toddlers and preschoolers are often afraid of monsters and other imaginary creatures, whereas older children are afraid of more realistic dangers, such as burglars or natural disasters.

Many bedtime fears can also be learned through simple conditioning. For example, the bedroom may be a source of anxiety for some children, especially if it is the place where the child is sent as punishment. Also, if the child has a nightmare or awakens distressed in the middle of the night, a parent typically comes into the room and turns on the light. Thus, a child may associate light with comfort and darkness with distress or nightmares.

What to Do If Your Child Is Afraid at Bedtime

Dealing with a child who is afraid of the dark or scared to go to bed at night is like walking a tightrope. It is a fine line between wanting to reassure him and not wanting to reinforce his fears by reassuring him too much. Ignoring his fears is cold and unfeeling. However, if you reassure him too much, you may subtly be giving the message that there is something to be afraid of. Most children outgrow their fears, but in the meantime here are some strategies you may want to try.

REASSURANCE. It is important to reassure children and let them know that they are safe. Let your child know that you are nearby and will make sure that nothing bad happens by saying things like "Mommy and Daddy are right downstairs and we'll always make sure that you are safe."

TEACH COPING SKILLS. Children need to be taught how to cope with frightening situations. Talk to your child about better ways to respond to fears, such as being brave or saying positive things, like "Monsters are just pretend." Discuss how you deal with something that you are afraid of. Read stories about children who are afraid and conquer their fears, such as *There's a Nightmare in My Closet* by Mercer Mayer. (For suggested stories on dealing with bedtime fears, see Appendix A, "Baby Bedtime Books.")

MONSTER SPRAY. Many families have found "monster spray" a wonderful way to help a child cope with bedtime fears. Take a spray-type bottle (be sure that it has not previously contained any chemicals such as plant food) and fill it with water. Some people add food coloring, but this can stain. Label it in large letters MONSTER SPRAY or BOGEYMAN SPRAY or whatever your child calls what he is afraid of. At bedtime, you or your child can spray the room to keep the monsters away. Keep the spray bottle next to the bed. During the night, if your child gets scared, he can spray the monsters away. This will give your child a way to cope and save you from having to come help him. However, note that some young children may view this as evidence that a monster actually exists!

USE YOUR IMAGINATION. Use your imagination to fight imaginary monsters. In addition to monster spray you can make up other things that will help your child. Logic isn't important. If it works, go with it. One family had a large old cat named Opus. They told their son, Jason, that Opus stayed up at night and made sure that everyone was safe. Opus also kept bogeymen away. So at bedtime they would bring Opus in, and their son would give him instructions to stay awake and guard the house. This satisfied their son. Opus, of course, would leave the room and go to sleep in his usual spot on the living room couch, but Jason felt safe believing that Opus was on patrol for bogeymen.

USE HUMOR. Provide your child with concrete coping skills. For example, make a nighttime announcement that will keep monsters away: "This is Sophie's mother. This house is officially declared a safe house. There are no monsters in this house."

HAVE FUN IN THE DARK. If your child is afraid of the dark, make being in the dark fun. For example, play flashlight tag or set up a treasure hunt for items that glow in the dark. Have a scavenger hunt for favorite toys using flashlights. Read in the dark by flashlight or candlelight. The more you make being in the dark fun, the less scary it will be for your child.

SECURITY OBJECTS. A security object, such as a favorite stuffed animal or blanket, can be reassuring to a child.

NIGHT-LIGHT. A low night-light often helps keep the monsters away. Leaving a bedroom door open may also help your child feel less isolated and afraid.

AVOID SCARY STORIES AND TELEVISION SHOWS. Avoid reading scary stories or watching scary movies. Remember, what may not seem frightening to you may be very frightening to a young child.

CHECK ON YOUR CHILD. Check on your child every five or ten minutes, so that your child has a predictable schedule of parental reassurance. This way your child will feel safe and secure, and won't have the need to call you.

SET LIMITS. At the same time that you are reassuring your child, you do need to set limits. Setting limits is necessary to prevent the behavior that your child exhibits when being scared from being reinforced. Checking closets and leaving a low night-light on is reasonable, but allowing your child to sleep with you every night may not be.

STAR SYSTEM. Some children receive reinforcement for being scared at night. They may be getting lots of attention or receiving special treats for being afraid. If this is the case, switch the scenario. Give your daughter lots of attention for dealing with her fears. Tell her how proud you are of her for being brave. Set up a star system: She earns stars for being brave and sleeping on her own. After earning a certain number of stars, she can turn them in for a treat, such as watching a favorite video, going to the park, or baking chocolate chip cookies with you.

RELAXATION TRAINING. You can also teach your child relaxation strategies to help her relax at bedtime and fall asleep. This will give her something else to think about while lying in bed, helping to distract her from her fearful thoughts. Also, it is impossible to be relaxed and scared at the same time. Our bodies simply do not work that way. So being relaxed will preempt being scared.

Relaxation strategies are presented in Chapter 9. These strategies are designed for adults but can easily be modified for children. For example, you can use guided imagery to help your child develop an image of a favorite relaxing place. Young children are also very successful at learning progressive muscle relaxation. For young children, modify the progressive muscle relaxation script provided in Chapter 9. Rather than simply telling your child to tense certain muscles, which can be a difficult concept for a youngster, use the images described in the box to help her tense her muscles.

NIGHTMARES

Nightmares are scary dreams that can wake your child, leaving him upset and in need of comfort. Many children are afraid to go back to sleep after a nightmare and often do not want to be left alone. Very young children do not know the difference between a dream and reality, so when they wake up, they do not understand that they were only dreaming and that the dream is now over. They may keep insisting that something scary that was about to happen in the dream is still about to occur. Your child may therefore be afraid and worried that something is still about to "get" him.

Many people ask whether young babies can have nightmares.

⭐ *Tensing Exercises for Muscle Groups* ⭐

Hands and arms—Squeeze a lemon in your hand.

Arms and shoulders—Pretend you are a furry, lazy cat who is stretching. Stretch your arms in front of you and over your head.

Legs and feet—You are walking through a big, squishy mud puddle. Squish your toes down into the mud and use your legs to help you push down to the bottom.

Stomach—Uh-oh, you are lying on the ground and a baby elephant is about to step on your stomach. Make your stomach hard so he won't crush you!

Stomach and chest—You have to squeeze through a very narrow fence, and you have to make yourself skinny. Suck in your stomach and hold your breath. Squeeze through that fence! Ah, you made it.

Shoulder and neck—Pretend you are a turtle and pull your head in tight by pushing your shoulders up to your ears. Hide your head!

Jaw—Bite down really hard on a big jawbreaker bubble gum.

Face—Try to get a pesky fly off your nose without using your hands. Wrinkle your nose and try to get him off. Oh, no. He's now on your forehead. Make lots of wrinkles and try to catch him between those wrinkles.

Adapted from A. S. Koeppen, "Relaxation Training for Children," *Elementary School Guidance and Counseling* 9 (1974): 14–21.

We really don't know. Given that they can't tell us whether or not they dream, there is no way to know whether they are having nightmares. By the second year of life, babies definitely dream and have nightmares. It is just difficult to know whether they have them younger than that.

What do young children have nightmares about? Most young toddlers have concerns about being separated from their parents and may have a nightmare about being lost or having something happen to a parent. Nightmares are more likely to happen following some difficult event in the child's life. For example, if your child has just started day care or if you have gone away overnight, your child is more likely to have a nightmare. For young children, nightmares may also be the reliving of a traumatic event, such as getting lost, getting a shot at the doctor's office, or being barked at by a big dog. By age two, nightmares begin to incorporate monsters and scary things that can hurt them.

Realize that nightmares are extremely common, with almost 75 percent of children having experienced at least one nightmare. One study found that 24 percent of children ages two to five years experience chronic nightmares, defined as having frequent nightmares for at least three months.

How to Avoid Nightmares

Not all nightmares can be avoided. They are a part of normal development and are a sign of your child's developing imagination. There are a few things you can do, however, to help reduce the likelihood of nightmares.

AVOID SCARY THINGS BEFORE BEDTIME. Don't read scary stories or watch scary movies immediately before bedtime. Don't play games that include your child's being chased by monsters or by the "big bad wolf." Don't play "I'm gonna get you."

ASSURE SAFETY. Be sure that your child understands that she is safe and that you are close at hand if she needs you. If she calls to you, be sure to respond quickly, especially following a nightmare. She will need this reassurance even more the next night after having a nightmare, so do respond to her needs.

REDUCE STRESS. If there is something in your child's life that you know is distressing, try to resolve it and reassure your child. If she is being bullied by a bigger kid at day care, talk to her day care provider. If she was recently bitten by a dog and has become terrified of dogs, work with her to help her get over her fear. Read stories about dogs. Visit a puppy. If your child suddenly experiences a significant increase in nightmares, try to evaluate why. Look for recurring themes that could give you a clue as to the cause, and then work to deal with the problem.

ENSURE ENOUGH SLEEP. After nights in which you don't get enough sleep, your body becomes sleep deprived or, more specifically, REM deprived. That is, your body needs REM sleep. When you don't get enough of it, your body will try to catch up the next night, and you will spend more time in REM sleep. Consequently, you will be dreaming more, and these dreams can often become more bizarre and scary than on other nights. So make sure that your child is getting enough sleep. This can help decrease the frequency and intensity of nightmares.

TALK ABOUT SCARY THINGS DURING THE DAY. Rather than talking about scary things at bedtime or during the night, wait until daylight hours. Otherwise, you may just scare your child more, making it harder to fall asleep.

ELIMINATE VITAMINS PRIOR TO BEDTIME. High-dose vitamins taken at bedtime can disturb sleep. Vitamins should not be taken at bedtime because they, along with some foods, can cause a person's metabolism to increase and result in nightmares. (Note, too, that some medications can also bring on nightmares.)

What to Do If Your Child Has a Nightmare

The best thing that you can do if your child has a nightmare is to comfort her. For babies and young toddlers, merely holding them and providing physical comfort is enough. For older toddlers and young children, verbal reassurance may also be needed. If your child is less than two years old, don't bother trying to explain the concept that "it was just a dream." She won't understand it. If your child insists on your putting a light on and leaving it on, that is okay. If you leave it on, put it on the dimmest setting possible so your child can fall back to sleep easily. Many children find a dim night-light that is left on all night to be reassuring. Also, having your child sleep with a security object or lovey can be helpful. For some children, this may be a stuffed animal or a special blanket. For others, it may be a family pet; even a fish in an aquarium will sometimes do.

Your child will have a hard time distinguishing between a dream and reality, so help your child understand that she is no longer in danger. You may also have to show your child that there are no monsters under the bed or in the closet. If she insists on checking whether her sibling or someone else is all right because she had a dream that that person was hurt, show her that the person is fine. (And don't be hurt if your child insists on the other parent for comfort. All children go through periods during which they want one or the other parent. This is an aspect of normal development that helps your child bond to both parents.)

With older children, you can have them draw pictures of their nightmare that they can then crumple up and throw in the trash. Dream catchers, which hang on the wall over a child's bed, can also help "catch" bad dreams. According to Native American legend, the hole in the center of the dream catcher allows good dreams to reach the sleeper, while the web catches the bad dreams. These types of symbolic gestures can be very comforting to a young child. Other strategies include having a child pretend he is watching a television set and have him "change the channel to a new dream" or telling him to flip his pillow over for a fresh start. Often these concrete suggestions can be very reassuring and will help make your child feel more in control.

Staying With Your Child

"My child doesn't want to be left alone after a nightmare. Should I stay with him? Is it okay if I bring him back to our bed?"

Parents often debate whether to allow their child to come into their bed and stay with them after a nightmare. This decision is a difficult one because you are trying to balance two different needs. On the one hand, you want to comfort your child, especially if he is terrified. On the other hand, you don't want to encourage him to join you in bed or give the message that it is okay to sleep with Mommy and Daddy (if it isn't okay with you).

Following most nightmares your child will be reassured by a few minutes of comfort. Stay with him in his room. Let him know that you are nearby and will make sure that he is safe and secure. Don't stay too long. Staying with him for a long time or allowing him in your bed can subtly reinforce the idea that there really is something for your child to be afraid of. If your child is clearly terrified, though, it is fine to let him stay with you. Be clear that you will stay with him or allow him into your bed only when he is sick or extremely frightened (again, only if you don't want your child in your bed every night). If not, you may find that your child has decided to have a "nightmare" every night.

Nightmares Versus Sleep Terrors

It is important to distinguish between a nightmare and a sleep terror (night terror) because they are two distinct entities and are dealt with differently. Nightmares usually occur in the latter part of the night, after several hours of sleep. Your child will recognize you and seek comfort from you. It may take her a while to fall back to sleep. She will also remember having the nightmare the next day. As you will recall from Chapter 13, sleep terrors occur within one to two hours of falling asleep. Your child will quickly return to sleep and will not remember the occurrence in the morning.

TEETH GRINDING

Lydia is ten months old. Her mother swears that Lydia grinds her teeth. She doesn't do it every night but enough that her mother has noticed.

A large number of babies grind their teeth—that is, what teeth they have. About 50 percent of all babies grind their teeth before they turn one year of age, with most starting between ten and eleven months. The sound of grinding teeth is unmistakable; you will know if your baby does it or not. But while the sound can be very loud and bothersome to you, there is nothing to be concerned about.

Teeth grinding, in medical jargon, is called "bruxism." Studies show that 70–90 percent of all adults grind their teeth to some degree, and about 5 percent do it often. It is also seen in children and adolescents. In babies, however, bruxism usually begins at about the age of ten months and occurs after the baby has her deciduous incisors (the two top front teeth and two bottom front teeth). Babies usually start to get their two bottom teeth at around six months, and by ten months have their two top teeth also. (Note, though, that it is not unusual for some babies not to have any teeth at all until they are a year old.) Babies can grind their teeth in any stage of sleep but are more likely to do it in non-REM sleep, especially stage two. This means that it is much more likely to occur in the first half of the night, although it can occur at any time. Some babies grind their teeth only sporadically, whereas others do it throughout most of the night.

While teeth grinding in adults can lead to dental problems, teeth grinding in babies is nothing to be alarmed about. It is highly unlikely that your child is doing any damage to her teeth. If you are worried, however, or see any changes in your child's teeth, be sure to consult a dentist. This behavior will eventually go away on its own.

ROCKING AND ROLLING

Henry is fifteen months old. Every night in his crib Henry rocks back and forth and bangs his head against the side of his crib. It drives his parents crazy. They often go into his room to tell him to stop banging.

This type of rocking and rolling is often seen in young children. It is officially called "rhythmic movement disorder." Every child is different in what he does, but it is usually some type of rocking, rolling, or head banging. Oddly, children find this a soothing way to fall asleep. Your baby may do this at naptime and bedtime to put himself to sleep. And remember that babies wake frequently during the night and need to put themselves back to sleep. Since your baby's head banging or rocking is his way of falling asleep, don't be surprised if this behavior occurs not only at bedtime but throughout the night. These rhythmic behaviors are similar to other ones that are often more recognized, such as sucking on a thumb or pacifier, rubbing the same spot on a blanket over and over again, or twirling hair (often Mom's).

Studies indicate that about two-thirds of nine-month-olds do some type of rhythmic behavior when they fall asleep, with about half stopping by eighteen months. At four years of age, fewer than one in ten children continue this behavior, but there are some people who continue these behaviors into adulthood. Body rocking is usually the earliest to start (around six months of age), followed by head banging and head rolling at nine to ten months. These behaviors are much more common in boys than in girls.

For most babies, head banging or body rolling is not problematic, but there are some children for whom it may be of concern. Some children who are developmentally disabled or autistic will repeatedly rock or bang their heads, and may hurt themselves. These children may require helmets or restraints to ensure that they do not injure themselves. Some children who are blind or have some neurological problem will also be more likely to be violent body rockers.

Head banging or body rolling does not mean, however, that your child has a neurological problem. If this is the only behavior that you have seen, and if your child is normal and healthy otherwise, you should not be concerned. If your child has a neurological or psychiatric problem, you will be aware of it from behavior during the day.

If your baby has no neurological or psychiatric problems, there is nothing much that you need to do. Babies often rock or bang their heads to fall asleep. This is normal. They will eventually stop. Also, don't worry about having to protect your child. Even if your child is banging his head voraciously, it is unlikely that he will hurt himself, so there is no need to put extra bumpers on the crib or place pillows in strategic places. Besides, it won't work. If a baby really wants to bang his head, he will do it no matter what creative tricks you try. Those children previously mentioned who require helmets are children who bang their head not as a soothing mechanism to fall asleep but as a way to injure themselves. This behavior is also exhibited during the day. This self-injurious behavior is substantially different from behavior exhibited as a way of falling asleep.

Be careful about reinforcing this behavior. If you go in to your baby every time he starts to rock or bang his head, you may be reinforcing his behavior without even realizing it. In that event he may be head banging to get your attention. If so, make sure that your child gets lots of attention from you during the day and ignore his head banging at night. You can occasionally look in on him at night, without waking him, to make sure he is okay.

For your own sake, move the crib or the bed away from the wall if the banging or rocking is keeping the rest of the family awake. If your child is in a bed rather than a crib, be sure to put guardrails on all sides before moving the bed so that he won't roll out of bed now that the wall is not there to act as a buffer. If the crib or bed is squeaking and keeping you awake, oil the screws and bolts. In addition, for safety reasons, frequently tighten all screws and bolts. Some children literally rock their crib or bed apart.

Finally, increase the amount of sleep your child is getting. Increasing naptimes and moving bedtime earlier may result in less sleep deprivation. Sleep deprivation often leads to more nighttime awakenings, when these behaviors occur.

There are other things that you can try, although they may not be very effective. Try putting a loud ticking clock or metronome in your child's room. The external rhythmic noise may help replace your child's need to bang his head or rock his body. If your child bangs his head against the side of the crib and is bruising himself, you can try putting him on a mattress on the floor. This may not always work; some children simply move closer to the wall and fall asleep there, banging away.

SLEEP STARTS

Valerie noticed that her three-year-old son, Michael, always jerked when he was falling asleep. His entire body would seem to jump right off the bed. She used to worry that these were some type of seizure until she began to notice that her husband seemed to have them as well.

Most people have experienced sleep starts, the common sensation of a sudden, often violent jerk of the entire body just as you fall asleep. Sleep starts are perfectly normal. Many people have the sensation that they are falling and then jerk back awake.

As you may recall from Chapter 2, sleep starts are caused by an intrusion of REM sleep. When you fall asleep at night, your body goes into non-REM sleep. Ninety minutes later, REM sleep occurs. For some reason, though, on some nights some people will have a few seconds to a few minutes of REM sleep right when they are falling asleep at night. This is called REM intrusion because REM sleep is intruding on a time when non-REM sleep should be occurring. REM sleep involves dreaming and paralysis of most of the body. Thus, the dream and the sensation of not being able to move make it seem as if you are falling, and then you jerk back awake. It doesn't mean anything other than perhaps that you are really tired. Some people have these sleep starts only when they haven't gotten enough sleep. Others have them every night.

In addition, some people naturally jerk when they are falling asleep. These are usually leg jerks, but the arms and other parts of the body can also jerk. Again, these are meaningless.

SLEEP TALKING

Sleep talking is formally called "somniloquy." Some people talk in their sleep all the time, while others do it rarely. Sleep talking is common and normal. It does not mean that there is a medical or psychological problem. Some people talk in their sleep. Some laugh. Some even moan.

Your child may do this fairly often. It is much more difficult to tell in babies whether they are babbling in their sleep or are just half awake. If your baby talks in her sleep, don't worry about it. Be entertained by it and otherwise leave it alone.

In older children and adults, sleep talking may occur during stressful periods, such as before the first day of school or during a stressful week at work. Don't be surprised by it and don't read too much into it. Some people believe that things spoken while sleeping come from the unconscious and are a window into the person's deepest thoughts and feelings. To date there is no empirical support for this theory.

Reminders

+ Bedtime fears are the most common fears of young children. There are ways to manage bedtime fears and teach your child to cope with these common fears.
+ Nightmares are scary dreams that can wake your child. There are ways to prevent nightmares and ways to deal with them.
+ There are other sleep behaviors common in young children, including teeth grinding, rocking to sleep, sleep starts, and sleep talking.

PART FIVE

"What About Me?": Adult Sleep and Sleep Problems

CHAPTER 15

"Now, I Can't Sleep!":
How Parents Can Get the Sleep They Need

Sarah is five months old and is finally sleeping through the night. The first few months were difficult, but Sarah has been sleeping well for the past three weeks. However, her mother, Deborah, still cannot sleep and is feeling run-down and exhausted. She has difficulty falling asleep and wakes frequently throughout the night. She thought that once Sarah was sleeping, all would return to normal, but that has not been the case.

All too often, even after the baby is finally sleeping through the night, parents continue to have sleep problems. There are also many other issues beyond babies that affect adults' sleep, including poor sleep habits, certain medications, and pregnancy.

THE BASICS OF SLEEP

"I Still Can't Sleep"

Many parents experience a delay in returning to normal sleep patterns once their baby is sleeping through the night, and it may take several months for them finally to sleep through the night.

The reason you, the parent, are having difficulty sleeping is probably because your body needs time to get back into old sleeping patterns. You have learned to wake frequently throughout the night along with your baby. You are probably still waking up at the times your baby used to wake up. You may even be going to check on the baby to make sure that she is really still asleep and that she's okay. Resist this urge. If she is awake and needs you, you will hear her. Your body simply needs time to return to your previous sleeping habits.

If you had problems sleeping before you were pregnant or had the baby, however, you will continue to have problems even after the baby is sleeping through the night. Be sure to read the tips that are provided later in this chapter, and read Chapter 16 to be sure that you don't have a sleep disorder that is affecting your sleep.

"I Feel Like a Zombie and I Can't Function"

As all too many parents know, not getting enough sleep has a major impact on their ability to function as parents, on the job, and as spouses. The bad news is that parents are more likely to be depressed, more anxious, and less satisfied in their marriages when they have a baby who doesn't sleep. The good news is that once the baby starts to sleep, parents feel better, are happier, and are more satisfied with their marriages.

Sleep Is Important

Sleep is not negotiable. Sleep is probably the most important thing that your body needs after food and water. Surprisingly, we don't really know why people need to sleep, but we do know what happens to people when they don't sleep. After just a few hours of sleep deprivation, a person's reaction time is slower and he is more likely to forget things and to become moody. After long periods of sleep deprivation, people begin to hallucinate—see things that are not there. Recent research has even shown that being partly sleep deprived over a period of time is equivalent to having a blood alcohol level of .10. In most states, a blood alcohol level of .08 is legally drunk (in other states it is .04). Basically, you cannot be a good parent, a good employee, or a good spouse if you don't get enough sleep.

Everyone needs about eight hours of sleep per night (yes, your grandmother was right). That is an average. Some people need nine or ten hours of sleep to feel their best. And, yes, there are some people who need only six or seven hours of sleep at night. But that is a rarity. When I worked in a sleep disorders center that treated adults as well as children, we never saw a person who got only six hours of sleep at night who was not sleep deprived. How can we tell that a person is sleep deprived? Careful analysis of sleep patterns reveals differences between normal sleep and the sleep of someone who is sleep deprived. For example, people dream more when they are sleep deprived, and they have different quantities of the different stages of sleep compared to when they are getting enough sleep.

But, you say, how can I get enough sleep when the baby is always crying, the laundry needs to be done, and the bills have to be paid? Well, this book has explained how to solve one major hurdle: getting your baby to sleep through the night. About the other things: First, *prioritize*. Then, *delegate*.

PRIORITIZE. This means figure out what is most important, what needs to be done, and what you can do without. Paying the bills is important; having a spotless house isn't. Having dinner is important; but having a full-course home-cooked meal isn't.

DELEGATE. You also don't have to do everything yourself. Your nine-year-old son can help by folding towels. They may not be folded exactly the way you would like, but that doesn't matter as long as it is done. Delegate your spouse, a friend, or a neighbor to call in a takeout order and pick it up on the way home from work. It may be worth it for a period of six months to hire people to do things that you would normally do. Get someone to come in and clean or do the laundry. Hire a local teenager to mow the lawn, rake the leaves, or even weed the flower beds. When people ask if there is anything that they can do to help, suggest something (whether it is picking up a gallon of milk at the store while they are there or watching the baby for a couple of hours).

This is not the time to be Superperson. People cannot do it all on their own. That is not realistic. Reality is that there is often too much to do and too little time in which to do it. So figure out what needs to be done and do what is important. And remember, sleep is important.

Napping

Babies are not the only ones who nap. Adults nap too. Napping is a universal behavior. In some cultures, napping is even the norm. Think of the Spanish siesta.

Naps are very important for parents of infants and toddlers, especially for parents of a baby less than three months old whose nighttime sleep is almost always interrupted. Naps are essential to make up for lost sleep. The rule of thumb is to nap when the baby naps. Even if you don't fall asleep, resting is beneficial. Although this may seem the perfect time to finally to get things done around the house or to make some phone calls, catching up on your sleep is probably more important.

Almost all naps occur at the same time every day, between noon and 5:00 p.m., that is about twelve hours after the midpoint of sleep the night before. So someone who slept from 11:00 p.m. until 7:00 a.m. will nap at 3:00 in the afternoon. Given this tendency for people to have what is apparently a twelve-hour rhythm, naps are likely to have a biological function. The average nap taken by adults lasts seventy minutes.

Naps can be very beneficial for daytime alertness but have two drawbacks. First, a person may feel groggy after waking from a nap. This typically involves a few minutes of disorientation when you may not be able to think clearly. For most of us that is not a problem, but for a physician on call or anyone else who is required to function immediately upon waking, it can be a serious issue. Second, naps can interfere with nighttime sleep, but this usually occurs only if the nap lasts longer than two hours or occurs too late in the afternoon.

Some people find that even a fifteen- to thirty-minute nap will make it harder for them to fall asleep at bedtime. That's because our sleep need builds during the day. If you nap, you will have less need to fall asleep at night. So if you sleep fine at night but just aren't getting enough sleep, a nap works well. However, for anyone who has trouble going to sleep or staying asleep, a nap may interfere with your ability to sleep at night. For this reason people with insomnia should avoid naps. For many, this becomes a vicious cycle—you don't sleep well at night, so you take a nap during the day, which makes it hard to sleep well the following night. It will take at least a few days to a week to break this cycle, forcing yourself to stay awake during the day to get your nighttime sleep back on track.

For some, napping that occurs at times other than mid-afternoon may be a sign of a sleep problem. For people with sleep apnea or narcolepsy, frequent daytime napping is a symptom of a sleep problem. People with a sleep disorder often nap at times other than during the afternoon and can nap many times in one day. Those with narcolepsy find short naps refreshing, whereas people with sleep apnea will still feel sleepy after a nap.

For others, especially parents of young children, naps are highly beneficial and may mean the difference between being able to function and not being able to function.

Making Up for Lost Sleep

Dan is the father of eight-month-old twins. During the week he usually goes to bed at midnight and has to get up for work at 6:30 a.m. If he is lucky, he sleeps the entire six and a half hours without being awakened by one of the twins. On weekends, he is able to sleep in and usually gets nine or ten hours of sleep. Despite getting all that sleep on the weekends, however, he is still tired.

Dan is finding that it is not easy to make up for lost sleep. One study showed that it takes at least three weeks to make up for lost sleep. Sleeping in on weekends will not solve the problem of not getting enough sleep during the week, nor will a one- or two-week vacation when you can sleep in each day. The box on the previous page will help you decide if you are getting enough sleep.

THE BEST WAY TO GET A GOOD NIGHT'S SLEEP

Here is a list of dos and don'ts for getting a good night's sleep.

+ **Maintain a regular daily schedule of activities.** Try to keep a set schedule during the day. Eat meals at the same times and plan your activities on a similar schedule.
+ **Sleep schedule.** Try to go to bed at the same time every night and wake up at the same time every morning. This will help regulate your body's inner clock. Sticking to the same schedule is important on weekends as well as on weekdays. It is best to go to bed within an hour of your usual bedtime. If you are having problems sleeping, avoid naps because they can interfere with nighttime sleep.
+ **Bedtime routine.** Bedtime routines are as important for adults as they are for children. Bedtime routines help your body know it is time to sleep before you even get into bed.
+ **Sleeping attire.** Wear loose-fitting, comfortable sleeping attire. Sexy lingerie may look great, but it won't help your sleep. The more comfortable you are, the better you will sleep.
+ **Exercise.** Exercise can help you sleep better. The best time to exercise is late afternoon or early evening, about five to six hours before bedtime. Avoid exercising within

four hours of bedtime because it will wake you up too much.

✦ **Relax.** Just prior to bedtime do something enjoyable and relaxing. Take a bath or read a good book. Don't pay your bills or choose that time to have an intense discussion with your partner. If you often worry at bedtime while you are trying to fall asleep, which is especially common for parents who are busy during the day, set aside a "worry time" earlier in the day.

✦ **Light snack.** Eat a light snack prior to bedtime if you are hungry. Going to bed hungry can interrupt your sleep. In addition, a cup of hot tea (decaffeinated, of course) or warm milk can help make you drowsy.

✦ **Your bedroom.** Make your bedroom as quiet and comfortable as possible. Have a good mattress and a pillow that you like. Make sure that the room is quiet. Running a fan or a "white noise maker" can help drown out sounds from the outdoors (this is not always best if it drowns out the sound of your baby if she needs you, although dampening the normal sounds your baby makes while sleeping can be helpful). A cool bedroom is better for sleep than a warm one. Also, a dark bedroom is best. It may be worth investing in room-darkening shades or blinds if your bedroom is too light. Finally, keep pets out of the bedroom, as they are notorious for jumping onto the bed and waking a person up (there was even a study published on the disruption of sleep by pets).

✦ **Can't sleep?** When you get into bed, turn off the lights (and the television!), close your eyes, and try to fall asleep. If you can't sleep, try to relax and rest as much as possible. Avoid looking at the clock and worrying about being tired the next day. This will just keep you awake longer. If you get frustrated, get out of bed and do something relaxing for twenty to thirty minutes and then return to bed when you feel tired and able to sleep. If you do get out of bed, try to avoid turning on bright lights that will wake up your brain even more.

+ **Sharing your bed.** If you share a bed with someone who is a snorer, a kicker, or a cover stealer, you may want to sleep elsewhere temporarily until you reestablish a better sleep pattern. If you think your bed partner has a sleep disorder, consult a physician.

+ **Avoid caffeine.** Avoid all caffeinated beverages after lunch. Note that many sodas, including Mountain Dew and some orange sodas, contain caffeine (see page 302 for a listing of caffeinated items). For example, Sunkist Orange has forty-two milligrams of caffeine per twelve ounces, whereas Diet Sunkist Orange has none. Check the ingredients listing on the label. Even chocolate and other foods with caffeine in them such as coffee yogurt or coffee ice cream can keep you up at night.

+ **Associate your bed with sleep.** Avoid doing other activities in bed other than sleep (and sex, of course). Don't eat in bed or pay your bills. Avoid even having a television in the bedroom (although I realize that this is an idea many people won't like). Learn to associate your bed and your bedroom with sleep.

+ **Avoid alcohol.** Avoid all alcoholic beverages. These interfere with sleep. They may help you to fall asleep more quickly, but they usually lead to your waking in the middle of the night.

THE EFFECTS OF DRUGS ON SLEEP

Many medications in use today may affect sleep. For example, antidepressants, a large class of drugs that are used to treat problems such as depression, anxiety, and pain, are also used to treat a number of sleep disorders. Each antidepressant affects sleep differently. The more traditional antidepressants, known as the tricyclic antidepressants, are amitriptyline (Elavil), imipramine (Tofranil), and desipramine (Norpramin). These medications are more likely to be sedating, decreasing night wakings and decreasing the time it takes to fall asleep. This is not true for all of them, though: some have no effect on sleep, and others can even increase wakefulness at night. Some antidepressants can make a person feel sluggish during the day. Because of this daytime sedating effect, many antidepressants are given as a single dose at bedtime.

The newer antidepressants, known as SSRIs (selective serotonin reuptake inhibitors), include fluoxetine (Prozac), paroxetine (Paxil), and sertraline (Zoloft). These medications are more likely to disrupt sleep, increasing how long it takes to fall asleep. However, they can also make you drowsy during the day. Newer SSRIs, such as citalopram (Celexa), are less disrupting to sleep. Other new antidepressants, including nefazadone (Serzone) and mirtazapine (Remeron), are even less likely to cause insomnia. In general, if you are taking a medication for depression, be sure to discuss with your doctor about its possible impact on sleep as well as daytime effects.

Benzodiazepines are drugs that are used for insomnia, anxiety, and seizure control, and as a muscle relaxant. Benzodiazepines usually have positive effects on sleep, including increasing total sleep time and decreasing night wakings. Commonly used benzodiazepines are alprazolam (Xanax), clonazepam (Klonopin), diazepam (Valium), lorazepam (Ativan), oxazepam (Serax), and temazepam (Restoril). Some benzodiazepines are longer acting than others. The longer-acting ones, if taken at bedtime, can cause a feeling of grogginess in the morning. Therefore, if you are taking these types of medications for sleep problems, you may need to try different ones to find the one that works best for you at night but leaves you awake and alert during the day. In addition, some of these drugs can make some sleep disorders worse. For example, benzodiazepines make sleep apnea worse and therefore can be dangerous for individuals who suffer from this disorder.

Other drugs that are used for anxiety, such as buspirone (BuSpar), clonidine (Catapres), hydroxyzine (Atarax, Vistaril), and propranolol (Inderal), can have variable effects on sleep. For example, buspirone can trigger restlessness. Also used to treat anxiety, as well as psychotic behavior and sleeplessness, are tranquilizers. Most tranquilizers are benzodiazepines, as discussed above. The most common tranquilizers are used for anxiety and include such drugs as Valium, Librium, and Xanax. These drugs can have some sedating effect and can help sleep. Be careful, however, because these drugs can also be addicting.

Steroids are a common treatment for many medical problems. The most common steroid used medically is prednisone; it is known to disrupt sleep and at higher doses can lead to nightmares. Common medications for cardiac problems, such as Inderal, Lopressor, and Visken, can cause difficulty falling asleep. These drugs also increase night wakings, and the resulting fragmented sleep can often lead to an increase in the number of dreams recalled. Bronchodilators for asthma can cause sleep disturbances also. Some have no effect on sleep, whereas others increase wakefulness.

Common over-the-counter medications can also affect sleep. For example, although antihistamines often cause drowsiness during the day, they can actually increase the time it takes to fall asleep at night. The newer antihistamines, such as Claritin, do not cause drowsiness. Appetite suppressants, which often contain a mild stimulant, can lead to insomnia, as you would expect. On the other hand, aspirin can be helpful for insomnia. Studies have shown that it can increase total sleep time and decrease night wakings. Some people report that aspirin works just as well for insomnia as some sleeping pills.

Caffeine, found as an ingredient in many foods and medicines, can lead to problems falling asleep at night. For those with restless legs syndrome or periodic limb movements in sleep (see Chapter 16), caffeine will make both of these conditions worse.

Caffeine

Caffeine can result in difficulties falling asleep and staying asleep.

Product	Serving Size	Caffeine Content (mg.)
SODA		
Coca-Cola	8 oz.	23
Diet Coke	8 oz.	31
Pepsi	8 oz.	25
Diet Pepsi	8 oz.	24
Dr Pepper/ Diet Dr Pepper	8 oz.	28
Mountain Dew/ Diet Mountain Dew	8 oz.	37
Sunkist Orange soda	8 oz.	28
Tab	8 oz.	47
Red Bull	330 ml.	80
COFFEE/TEA		
Cappucino	6 oz.	35
Coffee, decaf	8 oz.	5
Starbucks Coffee, grande	16 oz.	550
Starbucks Coffee, short	8 oz.	250
Starbucks Coffee, tall	12 oz.	375
Iced tea	8 oz.	25
Snapple iced tea (all kinds)	8 oz.	21
FOOD ITEMS		
Baker's chocolate	1 oz.	26
Chocolate milk	8 oz.	5
Dark chocolate, semisweet	1 oz.	20
Coffee ice cream	8 oz.	58
OVER-THE-COUNTER MEDICATIONS		
Dexatrim	1 tablet	200
Excedrin, max. strength	2 tablets	130
Nō-Dōz, max. strength; Vivarin	1 tablet	200
Nō-Dōz, regular strength	1 tablet	100

Alcohol also interferes with sleep. Although you may fall asleep more quickly after having a drink, it leads to middle-of-the-night wakings and earlier rising than you might prefer. Nicotine can cause difficulty falling asleep. Although many say that having a cigarette relaxes them, it may not help them to fall asleep at night.

Marijuana also affects sleep. Marijuana changes the duration of the different stages of sleep, and chronic use of the drug reduces REM sleep. After discontinuing its use, there is often REM rebound, meaning a significant increase in REM sleep to make up for the lost amount. This REM rebound will be experienced as a significant increase in dreaming.

Cocaine has a much more significant impact on sleep. Cocaine reduces the total amount of sleep the person obtains, especially REM sleep. Short-term withdrawal from cocaine produces significant changes in sleep, usually insomnia and fatigue.

It is important to evaluate whether any medication that you are currently taking is affecting your sleep. If you are taking any prescription medication, be sure to ask your physician or pharmacist what impact it may have on your sleep. Furthermore, it is important to stop many drugs slowly; for example, sudden withdrawal from benzodiazepines can be fatal. So be sure to ask your physician or pharmacist how to discontinue a drug safely if you wish to stop using it.

Sleeping Pills

In the past, sleeping pills often did more harm than good, especially for people whose only complaint was "I can't sleep" or "It takes me hours to fall asleep." There were a number of reasons that sleeping pills were *not* recommended:

+ Older types of sleeping pills affect the type of sleep you get. They modify the nervous system activity, which reduces REM sleep, the type of sleep when you dream.

+ The human body develops a tolerance to the older for-
mulations of sleeping pills after their repeated use. After
a while you have to take more and more to make you feel
sleepy.
+ You can experience rebound effects that cause a vicious
cycle. What often happens is that people take sleeping
pills for a while and then try stopping them. Usually,
though, the next two nights their sleep is very poor, so
they begin to take the pills again, convinced that they
need them. What is happening is that the body is experiencing rebound; it is actually going through withdrawal.
As a result, sleep will be worse for several nights. The
best thing to do is to wait two weeks after stopping taking
sleeping pills before evaluating your sleep.

A number of new hypnotics have come onto the market in the
United States. These medications are considered nonbenzodi-
azepines and work quite differently from the older sleeping medications. The two that have been out the longest are Ambien and
Sonata. Ambien works for a longer time, so should be taken only at
bedtime. Sonata works for a much shorter time, only about an hour,
so it can be taken at bedtime or in the middle of the night if you are
having difficulty falling back to sleep. Lunesta is a newer medication that works for an even longer time so that it will be helpful for
individuals who have difficulties both falling asleep and staying
asleep, with Indiplon likely to be on the market soon. Other new
sleeping medications will likely also be coming out soon, including
Ramelton and Gabitril. Both are in the final stages of drug testing
at the time of this writing. Tolerance is much less likely with these
newer sleeping medications. In the past, it was strongly recommended that none of these medications be taken for more than two
to three weeks; however, recent studies have found limited tolerance over six months and even a year for these medications, such as
Estorra and Ambien.

Before taking any sleeping medication, however, you should find out the reason for your sleeping problem and treat it appropriately. For example, if the reason that you are having problems falling asleep at night is because you have another sleep disorder such as sleep apnea, as discussed in Chapter 16, sleeping pills can make the problem worse. You can also become psychologically dependent on sleeping pills: if you are convinced that a sleeping pill is the only way you can get a good night's sleep, you won't be able to go to sleep without them.

Melatonin

There has been much in the news about melatonin and its impact on sleep. At this time melatonin is sold in health food stores under such names as Melatone. The reports state that ingestion of melatonin increases sleepiness. Some people have said that it is the new miracle cure—a way to treat insomnia and prevent jet lag.

Melatonin is naturally produced in the pineal gland and appears to be involved in the sleep process. Melatonin production in humans is highest between 10:00 p.m. and 3:00 a.m., and drops to low levels by 8:00 a.m. Thus, as melatonin increases, the need to sleep increases. The production of melatonin is influenced by exposure to light, whether it is daylight or artificial light. Light falls on the retina, which sends a message to the pineal gland. The argument is that if you take melatonin orally, you should get sleepy. However, there are mixed data about this phenomenon. Interestingly, people who have no functioning pineal gland (usually because of radiation treatment) continue to have good sleep patterns. That means that the pineal gland and melatonin production are only a small part of the sleep process. Sleep is much more complex.

Caution should be taken before using melatonin. Clinical studies need to be conducted to assess its effectiveness and any potential side effects. Studies so far have found little benefit of melatonin for sleep, other than for very specific reasons such as jet lag or shift work. Until melatonin is shown to be a sure thing, it is better to be safe than sorry. Moreover, although some argue that melatonin is a naturally produced substance and therefore shouldn't be of any harm, many naturally produced substances can be harmful. For example, insulin is a necessary chemical in the body, but too much insulin can be fatal. Lead, a natural substance, can cause brain damage. Also, since the Food and Drug Administration (FDA) does not regulate the manufacturing of melatonin, health food store supplies may be impure. A number of years ago L-tryptophan was the craze. L-tryptophan was supposed to help insomnia. But a batch of L-tryptophan, later believed to be contaminated, caused a serious blood disorder in a number of people. Before taking melatonin, therefore, check with your physician.

Should you put your child on melatonin? First, you should not give your child anything before checking with your pediatrician. Second, early studies on the effects of melatonin on baby rats showed that increased doses of melatonin can affect the development of the reproductive organs. Levels of melatonin are high in children prior to puberty. At the start of puberty, levels drop substantially. Thus, melatonin reduction may be an important aspect in the development of reproductive organs in adolescence. Therefore, giving a child or adolescent melatonin may have an impact on sexual development. Since no studies have been done to date on the long-term effects of melatonin in children, caution should be taken before administering it to your child.

SLEEP AND PREGNANCY

Stephanie is the mother of three-year-old twins, Ariel and Olivia. After several months of struggling, she has finally gotten the twins to go to bed by 8:30 and sleep through the night. However, Stephanie, who is now seven months pregnant, feels as though she never gets any sleep. She is up several times during the night to go to the bathroom, and at other times she is simply lying awake. She either can't find a comfortable position or is awakened when the baby starts to kick.

Each of the three trimesters of pregnancy is characterized by changes in sleep. Many women find that their sleep is disturbed throughout their pregnancy and that they are not getting a sufficient amount of sleep. This leads to feelings of fatigue during the day. If this is your first child, you may be able to catch up by napping during the day if your schedule allows. If you already have another child at home, however, especially one who doesn't sleep, it can be very difficult to cope. The following is an overview of what to expect during pregnancy as it relates to sleep.

First Trimester

Women often find that they are the most tired and sleep the most during the first trimester. High levels of the hormone progesterone during this period will make you feel sleepy and will increase the amount of sleep you need. You may be stunned to find yourself going to bed at 8:00 or 9:00 p.m. feeling that you can't keep your eyes open any longer, and not waking up until 8:00 the next morning. Given that this is a time of rapid development of the fetus, the woman's body is expending a great deal of energy and needs rest. Nighttime sleep also often becomes disrupted because of a need to urinate frequently. This need to urinate is caused by the enlarged uterus pressing on the bladder and by increased progesterone levels leading to increased urination. Taken together, these factors result in high levels of fatigue during the day and an increasing need for sleep at night. It is very common for women to find themselves napping during the day, even if they were never nappers before. If your schedule allows, give in to this increased need to sleep and don't try to fight it. Your body is sending you a message about what it needs.

Second Trimester

Sleep is much more normal during the second trimester. Development of the fetus has slowed down, so less energy expenditure is required by a woman. The need to urinate at night also diminishes because the uterus has moved from the pelvic region, where it presses on the bladder, to a position higher in the abdominal cavity, above the bladder. Women often report that they feel best during the second trimester.

Third Trimester

Sleeping becomes problematic again in the third trimester. The fetus is again going through a period of rapid growth, sapping much of the woman's energy. Pregnant women also tire more easily from carrying the weight of the larger fetus. Sleep is disrupted by backaches, frequent urination, heartburn, cramping of the legs, discomfort, and shortness of breath. Some women also find that the time when they are finally settling down for the night is when the baby decides to rev up. Women often complain that if the baby would just stop moving and kicking them in the ribs, they could get some sleep. The result of all of this is that women in the last trimester of pregnancy often take longer to fall asleep at night, are awake more frequently during the night, and take longer to fall back to sleep following waking. A study conducted in our laboratory found that by the end of pregnancy 97 percent of women report waking at night and 92 percent report restless sleep.

Additionally, pregnant women are more likely to develop other sleep disorders. Studies have shown that as pregnancy progresses, women are apt to begin snoring and develop sleep apnea (see Chapter 16). After the twentieth week of pregnancy, restless legs syndrome (RLS) may develop, also interfering with the ability to fall asleep at night. Leg cramps may also interrupt sleep, with 75 percent of women reporting them in their third trimester. Leg cramps may be related to low calcium or low potassium levels.

Reminders

+ Many adults have sleep problems.
+ To combat sleep problems, make sleep a priority in your life and develop good sleep habits.
+ Common drugs and medications can affect your sleep.
+ Sleep during pregnancy can be problematic.

CHAPTER 16

"I'm So Tired":
Common Adult Sleep Disorders

"The baby is finally sleeping, but now my husband's snoring is keeping me up!"

The problem of adult sleep disorders is as common as those seen in infants and toddlers. Unfortunately, while an estimated 40 million adults suffer from chronic sleep disorders, fewer than 5 percent of these individuals have their problem diagnosed and treated. Common adult sleep disorders include sleep apnea, insomnia, restless legs syndrome, periodic limb movements in sleep, and narcolepsy.

DO YOU HAVE A SLEEP DISORDER?

This can be a difficult question to answer. Most people do not realize that they have a sleep disorder, or they believe that it is simply the way they are. To determine whether you may have a sleep disorder, ask yourself the following questions: Do you have problems falling asleep at night or staying asleep? Are you sleepy during the day? If you answered yes to either of these two questions, you may have a sleep disorder. But first you need to be sure that you are getting enough sleep or at least trying to get enough sleep. To be sure, you need to be in bed at least eight hours at night. If you are not in bed for an adequate number of hours every night, you need first to try to get enough sleep. If you are getting enough sleep and are still having problems sleeping or are sleepy during the day, then you may be suffering from a sleep disorder. The only way to know if you have a problem is to be evaluated at a sleep disorders center. To find an accredited sleep disorders center near you, contact the American Academy of Sleep Medicine at (708)492-0930 or log on to their Web site at www.aasmnet.org.

WHICH SLEEP DISORDER DO YOU HAVE?

Again, the best way to know which sleep disorder you have is to be evaluated by a trained sleep specialist at a sleep disorders center. An overnight sleep study (see below for a complete explanation) may also be necessary to diagnose your problem. Without a sleep study it may not be possible to identify the problem or the severity of the disorder. It would be like not having blood test results if a doctor suspects that you are anemic. You cannot know without the definitive results.

ASSESSMENT OF SLEEP DISORDERS

A thorough evaluation for a sleep disorder involves a number of steps. The first step is an extensive interview during which the doctor will gather information about your sleep history. The doctor will probably ask you every possible question about your sleep: what time you go to bed, how long it takes you to fall asleep, whether you wake up during the night, what time you wake up in the morning, any naps that you take, and any behaviors that occur in your sleep, such as snoring, restless sleep, and sleep talking. If the doctor suspects a specific sleep disorder, you will be asked extensively about typical symptoms experienced (these will be discussed shortly). If you share a bed with someone, that person may also be asked some questions. For example, you may not be aware that you snore or talk in your sleep.

You will also be asked a number of questions that are indirectly related to sleep. For example, you will be questioned about evening activities such as television watching and bedtime routines, about what occurs during a typical day—such as daytime sleepiness, meals, and caffeine intake—and about feelings of anxiety and depression. A complete medical history will also be taken, which will include questions about major illnesses and hospitalizations, any medications that you are currently taking, and your overall health.

The second step in the evaluation of sleep problems is to keep a sleep diary. A typical sleep diary includes information on what time you went to bed, how long it took you to fall asleep, how often and how long you were awake during the middle of the night, what time you woke up in the morning, your total sleep time, and the length and time of naps. You will likely be asked to keep sleep diaries for at least two weeks, but possibly longer. It is important that these diaries be accurate, as they help to diagnose your problem and to assess whether any prescribed treatments are working.

In cases where there is a concern about an underlying physiological problem such as sleep apnea or periodic limb movements in sleep (PLMS), the doctor is likely to schedule a polysomnography (PSG). A PSG usually involves sleeping overnight at a sleep center, although sometimes these tests are conducted at home. If you are to stay overnight at a sleep center, you will be asked to arrive two to three hours prior to your normal bedtime. A technician will tape or glue to your skin a number of sensors and monitors that will measure heart rate, breathing rate, leg movements, eye movements, and brain waves. These measurements will help evaluate when you fall asleep, the stages of sleep you are in, and whether or not you have a sleep disorder. You will also be monitored all night by a technician, and your sleep will be recorded by an infrared video camera. "How in the world am I going to sleep?" you may ask. Surprisingly, almost everyone sleeps, although some people feel that they do not get as much sleep as usual.

In addition to a PSG, you may undergo a multiple sleep latency test (MSLT). This test, which is performed the day following the overnight study, will evaluate your level of sleepiness during the day. The MSLT consists of four or five twenty-minute naps taken at two-hour intervals. So if you wake up in the morning at 8:00 a.m., you will be asked to lie down and try to fall asleep at 10:00 a.m., noon, 2:00 p.m., and 4:00 p.m. The test measures how long it takes you to fall asleep. If you fall asleep, you will be awakened after fifteen to twenty minutes. If you do not fall asleep, you will be asked to get out of bed after twenty minutes.

After obtaining all of the above information, a diagnosis will be made and a treatment plan developed.

Below is an overview of the most common and most disruptive sleep disorders experienced by adults. You should realize, though, that there are more than eighty different sleep disorders, and therefore the sleep problem you are experiencing may not be one of those discussed below.

SNORING

"*My* husband's snoring is driving me crazy. What causes it and what can he do?"

Snoring occurs only when a person is asleep. It is caused by the flapping of the airway muscles, which tend to vibrate during sleep once the muscles of the neck become relaxed. Most snoring occurs when the person is inhaling.

Snoring can be incredibly loud. Just ask anybody who lives with a snorer. To give you some perspective, loud snoring may reach eighty decibels. Normal speech is only forty decibels. A baby crying is about sixty decibels. Eighty decibels is similar to a large dog barking. Some people's snoring is so loud that the noise they generate exceeds government standards for noise in the workplace.

Men are twice as likely to snore as women. This may be related to a protection factor by female hormones. After menopause, when female hormone production diminishes, women are just as likely to snore as men. About 25 percent of all men snore, and the likelihood of snoring increases with age. By middle age (forty-one to sixty-five), almost 60 percent of men snore. The most likely reason why snoring becomes more prevalent as people get older is a loss of muscle tone in the muscles of the throat.

Several factors contribute to snoring. First, someone with a small airway (caused by enlarged tonsils or a large neck) is more likely to snore. Many overweight people snore because obesity leads to a constriction of the airway. A second common contributor is mouth breathing. People who snore almost always breathe through their mouths during sleep. Third, a number of drugs and medications can lead to snoring. Sleeping pills, alcohol, and other sedatives all can relax the muscles in the area of the throat, causing an increase in snoring. Allergies and colds can lead to snoring, since nasal congestion can force the person to breathe through his mouth.

Snoring should not be ignored. Some people believe that snoring is a sign of being a "good sleeper." This is absolutely not true. Snoring isn't normal, and people shouldn't snore. For some people snoring isn't harmful, although it can cause problems for other people in the household. Many couples sleep in separate bedrooms because one person's snoring chases the other out of the bedroom. For others, however, snoring can actually be a symptom of a more serious sleep disorder, sleep apnea (which is discussed below). One way to tell if a person who snores has sleep apnea is to determine if the person has daytime sleepiness. People with sleep apnea are very sleepy during the day. A snorer who isn't very sleepy may be just a snorer.

Even if the snoring is not affecting the person's health, treatment may still be sought, especially on the encouragement of the bed partner who isn't getting any sleep. There are hundreds of devices available that claim to stop snoring. Most try to keep the mouth closed or open the nasal airway. Such devices include bandages that go over the nose (such as Breathe Right) or prongs that widen the nose. Other devices try to keep the sleeper off his or her back, since many people snore only when on their back. An easier and cheaper alternative is simply to sew a pocket onto the back of a pajama top or T-shirt and place a tennis ball in it. Other more elaborate and expensive methods include alarms that go off when the person rolls onto his or her back.

There are some excellent dental devices that help prevent snoring. Be careful about substituting an athletic mouth guard for a proper dental device because these may result in difficulty breathing. For some, snoring is so bad that they opt for surgery. The two most common surgical techniques include the removal of the tonsils and adenoids or a uvulopalatopharyngoplasty (UPPP), which removes much of the tissue in the airway.

SLEEP APNEA

Steve is forty-four years old and has been snoring for ten years. His snoring has gotten much worse over the past two years, and now many nights his wife ends up sleeping in the guest room because his snoring is so loud. His wife says that many times throughout the night Steve seems to stop breathing. In the morning he often wakes up with a headache, which goes away after a few hours. Even after getting eight hours of sleep at night, Steve still feels terrible during the day. He is always sleepy and feels lethargic. He often naps during his lunch hour.

Steve is a classic example of someone who has sleep apnea, a disorder in which a person has repetitive episodes of upper airway obstruction during sleep. This means that numerous times throughout the night a person stops breathing because his airway closes. These events cause frequent arousals and awakenings during the night. To receive a diagnosis of sleep apnea, someone must stop breathing at least 5 times per hour. However, most stop breathing many more times than that. For example, there are some people who stop breathing more than 150 times per hour. Basically, these people can't sleep and breathe at the same time.

The concern many people have about apnea is that they are going to die in their sleep. This will not happen. The body is incredible. Immediately after the person stops breathing, the brain will tell the body to wake up, and breathing will resume. The more immediate concern is the excessive sleepiness that occurs during the day and the dangers that can go along with it, such as falling asleep while driving. A more long-term concern is that the individual is at much greater risk for heart disease and early death. Basically, the body does not react well to repeated lapses in breathing.

The typical person with sleep apnea is an overweight middle-aged man, but many others develop sleep apnea. Women get sleep apnea but are much more at risk for it after menopause. Thin people also get sleep apnea. But even though weight is often a determining factor, the heaviest person may not have sleep apnea, whereas the skinniest person may.

Symptoms of Sleep Apnea

Some people will have all of the symptoms listed below, whereas someone else will have only a few. Most people with sleep apnea don't even know that they have a problem. Usually it is the bed partner who suspects a problem or is so bothered by it that he or she forces the person to seek help.

+ **Snoring.** Most adults with sleep apnea snore. Not all snorers, though, have sleep apnea. When the muscles of the airway relax during sleep, they have a tendency to flap (like a sail not pulled taut in the wind). Snoring is the sound of the muscles flapping. Most people with sleep apnea snore every night and throughout the night. Snoring is more likely to occur when lying on the back, but can occur in any sleep position. Many people are not even aware that they snore unless others tell them (including the neighbors). Others snore so loud that they even wake themselves.
+ **Breathing pauses.** Sleep apnea is characterized by breathing pauses. A person will stop breathing anywhere from just a few seconds to, at the most, forty-five seconds. To start breathing again the person must first wake up.
+ **Daytime sleepiness.** The one symptom that is almost universal to sleep apnea, and often the only one these individuals are aware of, is daytime sleepiness, caused by the numerous arousals throughout the night. It is almost like being awakened by your baby every five minutes throughout the entire night. People with sleep apnea may be so sleepy that they fall asleep during sex, while driving, and even in the midst of conversations.
+ **Coughing and choking during sleep.** Some people with sleep apnea find that they wake up during the night coughing and choking.

✦ **Dry mouth.** Many people with sleep apnea wake up with a dry mouth because they are breathing and snoring with their mouth open.

✦ **Morning headaches.** Another common symptom of sleep apnea is a headache in the morning, caused by the decrease in oxygen to the brain throughout the night. Usually by midmorning the headache has gone away.

✦ **Restless sleep.** Because of the frequent arousals throughout the night, a person with sleep apnea often appears to be a restless sleeper. With each arousal the person may move his legs or turn over. In addition, the person may find his bedcovers are all over the bed when he wakes in the morning.

Other common symptoms include:

✦ **Insomnia.** Surprisingly, some people with sleep apnea complain of insomnia. Although they are extremely sleepy and tired, they are unable to fall asleep at night. This is because they stop breathing as they are falling asleep. When the breathing pause occurs, they have an arousal and wake up. The "insomnia" is, thus, caused by the breathing problems.

✦ **Impotence.** Impotence can be related to sleep apnea in some men. Once the apnea is treated, the impotence problems often go away.

✦ **Daytime problems.** Another common complaint of people with sleep apnea is that they don't feel that they function well during the day. They may become forgetful. They may feel irritable, anxious, or depressed.

Treatment of Sleep Apnea

A number of treatment options are available for sleep apnea. The best treatment for you will depend on the severity of your sleep apnea, what is contributing to your symptoms, and what will work best for you. Some of these treatments are similar to those mentioned above for snoring.

CONTINUOUS POSITIVE AIRWAY PRESSURE (CPAP). For most people with sleep apnea, CPAP is the treatment of choice. CPAP is a machine that has a mask attached to it. The purpose of CPAP is to keep the airway open so that normal breathing can occur. The CPAP machine generates air pressure, and this air pressure is forced down the nose, causing the airway to stay open. CPAP machines can be set at different pressures. An overnight test will need to be conducted at a sleep center to find a pressure that is optimal for you: one that gets rid of snoring, decreases apnea, and does not interfere with your sleep. Many insurance companies will pay for CPAP as part of your medical coverage.

SURGERY. There are a number of surgical options available to treat sleep apnea. In some instances the removal of the tonsils and/or adenoids can be effective. This surgery is usually done on children with sleep apnea and is the treatment of choice for them. In adults, this procedure is performed if it is clear that the person's tonsils or adenoids are enlarged and are obviously contributing to the problem. It is generally effective if the person has very mild apnea, but it may also benefit some cases of moderate to severe apnea. An ear, nose, and throat (ENT) specialist will evaluate you for this type of surgery.

For some individuals, sleep apnea is caused by a severely deviated septum (that is, the wall that divides the nasal passages is crooked), and surgery to correct this abnormality can solve the problem. An ENT doctor also will provide expertise in this area.

A surgery that has become common in the treatment of sleep

apnea is called a uvulopalatopharyngoplasty, otherwise known as a UPPP. This surgery, typically done by laser, removes excess tissue in the airway, including the tonsils. This widens the opening of the airway so that no obstructions occur, and the person can breathe normally while sleeping. This surgery can be conducted on an out-patient basis, but it does not work for everyone. It works best for those with mild to moderate sleep apnea and is effective in about 50–70 percent of individuals.

DENTAL APPLIANCE. Some people with mild to moderate sleep apnea benefit from a dental appliance. Similar to that used for people who grind their teeth in their sleep, this appliance is worn at night, and it moves the lower jaw slightly forward. Moving the jaw forward helps keep the airway open and will decrease both snoring and sleep apnea. The use of a dental appliance on a nightly basis does not cause any jaw problems, which is a common concern. A dentist or orthodontist usually fits this device, which can be expensive. Unfortunately, many medical insurance plans will not cover the cost.

WEIGHT LOSS. Weight is often a contributor to sleep apnea. For some people a difference of even five pounds can increase or decrease sleep apnea. Five pounds less, and the sleep apnea goes away. Five pounds more, and it comes back. For these people simple weight loss can solve the problem. For people who are more overweight, weight loss will help decrease apnea, and enough weight loss may also eliminate the problem. In the meantime, however, additional treatments are recommended.

SLEEP POSITION. For those people who snore and have apnea only when sleeping on their back, sleeping in any other position will often treat the problem. There are many devices on the market that are geared toward preventing people from sleeping on their back. The easiest solution, however, is to sew a pocket onto the back of a pajama top or T-shirt and place a tennis ball in it. Then, when you roll onto your back and get jabbed by the tennis ball, you will roll back over onto your side or stomach. This easy solution can solve the problem for some people.

MEDICATION. If allergies or nasal congestion cause your sleep apnea, drugs that reduce these symptoms can help you sleep. Although over-the-counter medications can help, it is best to discuss these problems with your doctor.

What Not to Do

First of all, sleep apnea is a serious problem that should not be ignored. Unfortunately, many people do ignore it because they don't know they have it or discount it, since they think "everyone snores." However, it is important to avoid certain courses of action.

+ **Don't take sleeping pills.** If you are having a difficult time falling asleep, you may be inclined to take a sleeping pill. This could backfire on you. Sleeping pills can make sleep apnea significantly worse because the medication will even further relax the muscles that you use to breathe. The more relaxed the muscles, the worse sleep apnea will be. Therefore, sleeping pills can be dangerous and can cause you even more sleeping problems.
+ **Exercise caution when using any form of sedative, tranquilizer, antihistamine, or painkiller.** If you think that you have sleep apnea and are taking these types of medications for anxiety, allergies, or pain, be sure to discuss this with your doctor. These medications may make your sleep apnea worse.
+ **Avoid alcohol.** Alcohol is sedating and makes sleep apnea worse. Not only does alcohol increase sleep apnea, but it also interferes with sleep. Although alcohol may help a person fall asleep faster, it can lead to waking in

the middle of the night and early-morning rising. It also makes a person's sleep lighter, with less deep sleep than is needed.

✦ **Reduce caffeine intake.** Caffeine is a stimulant that can interfere with falling asleep. However, for many people, caffeine becomes part of a vicious cycle. These people are sleep deprived from the sleep apnea, leading to daily sleepiness. They take caffeine to stay awake, which makes it more difficult to fall asleep the next night. The cycle then continues the next day and the next. In the long run, if the sleep apnea is treated, the sleepiness and need for caffeine will be reduced.

INSOMNIA

For the past few years Caroline has been having problems falling asleep at night. Every night she gets into bed at 11:00. She then tosses and turns until about 12:30, when she finally gets frustrated and goes downstairs to watch television. She usually returns to bed at about 1:00, finally falling asleep between 2:00 and 3:00. When her alarm goes off at 7:15, she feels as if she could sleep for another few hours. She says that she walks around like a zombie all day, both looking forward to and dreading going to bed again that night.

Insomnia usually begins during a person's late twenties or early thirties. Many people suffer for years before seeking help, and many simply treat themselves by using drugs or alcohol to help them sleep at night and by drinking a great deal of caffeine during the day to combat their sleepiness.

Symptoms

There are two primary symptoms of insomnia.

✦ **Difficulty sleeping.** People with insomnia have problems sleeping: trouble falling asleep at night, waking in the middle of the night, or waking up too early in the morning and not being able to return to sleep.

✦ **Daytime fatigue.** The result of not getting a good night's sleep is being tired during the day. This can lead to a significant impact on daytime functioning at home, on the job, and socially. Although people with insomnia often feel fatigued, they usually are not excessively sleepy.

Other symptoms include:

✦ **Effects on mood.** Many people with insomnia feel depressed or anxious. They may be irritable and have little energy.

✦ **Decreased attention and concentration.** As a result of the sleep deprivation caused by insomnia, some people will have problems with concentration at work or at school, especially when listening to a lecture or in a meeting.

What Causes Insomnia?

Insomnia can have many different causes, which makes it different from the other sleep disorders discussed. Again, it is important to understand that not all people who have problems sleeping actually have insomnia. Many other sleep disorders, such as sleep apnea and restless legs syndrome, interfere with a person's ability to fall asleep and thus are experienced as insomnia. For those who do have insomnia that is not the result of another sleep disorder, it can be the result of many factors. For example, some people have insomnia as the result of anxiety or depression. However, most people's insomnia is learned. Something happens that interferes with a person's sleep, whether it is the birth of a baby, illness, pain, or shift work. Once the sleep becomes disturbed, it continues to be problematic because there is a continued association between sleeplessness and situations and behaviors that are associated with sleep, such as lying in bed. Then lying in bed where you just spent several sleepless nights will cause you to feel tense and frustrated. These feelings will make it even more difficult to fall asleep. Once the pattern is established it can continue for months or years. Also, poor sleep habits often develop, such as spending too much time in bed, not keeping to a consistent bedtime and wake time, and napping during the day.

An additional problem can be negative thoughts about sleep and being unable to fall asleep. This is experienced by many insomniacs and also leads to a vicious cycle: the more you try to sleep, the more agitated you will become, and the less likely you will be able to fall asleep. Trying too hard to fall asleep can simply add to the problem. Also, thoughts such as "I'll never be able to fall asleep" contribute to the problem.

Treatment

The best treatment for insomnia depends on what is causing the problem. For example, if the problem is a result of depression or anxiety, then the best treatment is psychotherapy or medication, such as an antidepressant or antianxiety drug. In addition, it is important to determine whether another sleep disorder, such as sleep apnea or restless legs syndrome, is causing you to have problems falling asleep. What feels like insomnia to you may actually be another problem. If this is the case, treating the actual sleep disorder will cure the problem.

If your insomnia is not caused by depression, anxiety, or another sleep disorder but involves some other disturbance of your normal sleep routine, there are two primary options.

MEDICATION. Many people try medication for insomnia. Some of the more common ones are Ambien and Sonata. A newer choice is Estorra, with several other sleeping medications about to be sold in the United States. These medications have been found to have few negative effects, and recent studies indicate little tolerance over long periods, whereas in the past, it was recommended that sleeping medications not be taken for more than two to three weeks. Drugs to help you sleep at night may not always be a good long-term solution, however (see Chapter 15 for why drugs are not always the answer).

STANDARD TREATMENT FOR INSOMNIA. Research has shown that standard cognitive-behavior therapy is the most effective treatment for insomnia. Study after study has shown that if you diligently follow the seven rules outlined in the box below, you can successfully fall sleep and stay asleep.

In addition, there are other things that you can try to help you sleep better.

+ **Relaxation.** Research has shown that relaxation training is effective in 45 percent of cases. You can learn to relax using a number of different techniques, including progressive muscle relaxation, guided imagery, and meditation. Several methods are covered in Chapter 9. There are also several good books available to teach you ways to relax.

+ **Hot bath.** A twenty-minute hot bath taken an hour or two before bedtime can often help you to sleep. The hot bath affects body temperature, which makes you tired and helps to prolong deeper natural sleep. Be careful about hot baths if you have any circulatory disorders. If this is the case, consult your physician first.

Seven Rules for Beating Insomnia

1. **Choose a set wake-up time.** Wake up at exactly the same time every day, no matter how much sleep you got the night before.
2. **Choose a bedtime.** Choose the earliest possible bedtime that enables you to get the sleep you need. However, too much time in bed will lead to lighter, more interrupted sleep, so an appropriate bedtime is one that enables you to get the sleep that you need but doesn't let you be in bed too long. You only want to spend the amount of time in bed that you actually need for sleep.
3. **Go to bed when you are sleepy, but not before your chosen bedtime.** Don't go to bed until you are sleepy. So if you are still wide-awake at your chosen bedtime, wait a while longer until you are sleepy enough to fall asleep quickly.
4. **Get out of bed when you can't sleep.** If you are lying in bed and can't sleep, get out of bed and do something relaxing out of the bedroom. Read a book, watch television, or do something else relaxing; then go back to bed when you feel sleepy enough to fall asleep quickly. Again, if you do not fall asleep quickly, get up. Keep repeating this cycle until you fall asleep. You need to get out of bed when you can't sleep both at bedtime and in the middle of the night.
5. **Don't worry or plan in bed.** When lying in bed at night, don't spend the time worrying or planning for the next day. Set aside another time of the day to do these things. If you automatically start thinking and worrying when you get in bed, get up and don't head back to bed until your thoughts won't interfere with falling asleep. Thinking in bed is a habit, and one that you can break.

6. **Use your bed for sleep only.** Don't do anything but sleep in your bed. That is, don't do other activities, such as eat, watch television, or pay bills in your bed. (Sex is allowed.)
7. **Avoid naps.** Naps will interfere with your ability to fall asleep at bedtime, so no naps.

✦ **Keep a strict sleep schedule.** It is best to maintain a strict sleep schedule in which you go to bed at the same time every night and wake up at the same time every morning.

✦ **Don't stay in bed too long.** One problem that people often have is staying in bed too long. Don't stay in bed nine or ten hours if you need only eight hours of sleep. It is better to be in bed only the exact number of hours that you need sleep. This is called sleep restriction. It will consolidate your sleep, especially if you have long periods of being awake in the middle of the night or wake too early in the morning. To do this, you will need to keep a sleep diary to determine how much you actually sleep. Many people believe that they sleep less than they actually do. By keeping a sleep diary for two weeks you can figure out the average amount of time you sleep per night. Then for the first five to seven days limit the time you are in bed each night to the average number of hours that you actually slept for the past two weeks. Once you are sleeping the entire time that you are in bed, gradually increase the amount of time that you allow yourself to sleep. Increase this time by small amounts, anywhere from fifteen to thirty minutes. This method will help consolidate your sleep and will help you associate your bed with sleep. This process can take from a few days to several months to accomplish. The one side effect that you need to be aware of is that you may be sleepy during the day from the initial sleep deprivation.

Don's sleep diaries showed that he was going to bed at 11:00 every night but not falling asleep until 12:30. He would then wake at 7:00 every morning. He averaged six and a half hours of sleep every night. To start sleep restriction, he limited himself to being in bed only six and a half hours a night for one week. By the end of that week he was sleeping the entire time he was in bed. He then gradually increased the amount of time that he was in bed, starting with six hours and forty-five minutes and adding fifteen minutes every few nights. It took him several weeks to get to the eight hours that he believed he needed, and he found that he was now falling asleep quickly and sleeping the entire time he was in bed.

+ **Reduce alcohol and drug use.** Alcohol and drugs interfere with sleep. For someone with a drug or alcohol problem, withdrawal can occur in the middle of the night, causing the person to wake. Reducing or eliminating alcohol and drug use is beneficial to combating insomnia.
+ **Watch the clock and stay up as long as possible.** Some people get caught in a vicious cycle of trying without success to fall asleep and then becoming frantic. Being frantic does not help falling asleep. If this is true for you, simply watching the clock and trying to stay awake as long as possible will break this pattern. Do this for a few nights in a row, and you will learn that you can still function the next day with less sleep than you would want. You will also decrease the worry when you can't fall asleep on other nights. This suggestion, while it seems to counter

all the other advice provided in this book, can be helpful for some, but it may not work for all.

✦ **Sleep hygiene.** Keep good sleep hygiene. Chapter 15 provides a list of the best dos and don'ts for getting a good night's sleep.

RESTLESS LEGS SYNDROME AND PERIODIC LIMB MOVEMENTS IN SLEEP

Two sleep disorders that are often related are restless legs syndrome (RLS), which interferes with falling asleep, and periodic limb movements in sleep (PLMS), which can also interfere with going to sleep but primarily leads to frequent wakings during the night. Both of these also often lead to daytime sleepiness.

Restless Legs Syndrome (RLS)

RLS is characterized by an uncomfortable "crawling" feeling in the legs, usually below the knee, when the person lies down to go to sleep. This uncomfortable feeling is alleviated by moving the legs while still in bed or leaving the bed to walk or pace. Unfortunately, the symptoms return when you stop moving. The result is difficulty falling asleep and insomnia. This feeling is often difficult to describe, but some people say that it is like "worms crawling" or that it is "creepy-crawly," or they use words like "prickling," "tickling," and "itching." In addition, RLS symptoms can occur at any time of the day, resulting in problems when sitting for long periods, such as at the movies or on long car rides. No one knows what exactly causes RLS, although in some people it is related to a deficiency of iron or low levels of folic acid. It is also not known why some people have RLS symptoms one night and not another.

RLS is relatively common, affecting between 5 and 15 percent of adults. RLS can be associated with pregnancy (up to 15 percent of pregnant women have RLS, which usually appears after the twentieth week). About 80 percent of individuals with RLS also suffer from PLMS (although the opposite is not always true).

Periodic Limb Movements in Sleep (PLMS)

PLMS is a condition in which a person's limbs, usually the legs, repetitively jerk or kick during sleep. If you have this disorder, you may complain that your legs often jerk, and anyone who shares your bed will report that you kick in your sleep. People with PLMS often find that they are restless sleepers, and their bed is often a mess in the morning. These people typically complain of insomnia, either because they can't fall asleep or because they wake frequently. PLMS is similar to apnea in that people with these disorders often are unaware of their problem, other than the resulting daytime sleepiness and/or insomnia that may result. As with RLS, PLMS may be related to an iron deficiency or low levels of folic acid. But for most people there is no clear reason for the sleep disorder.

Although we don't know exactly how many people have PLMS, we do know that the prevalence increases with age. For example, 44 percent of individuals over the age of sixty experience PLMS compared to 5 percent of those between thirty and fifty years.

Treatment

For those people whose RLS or PLMS is related to an iron deficiency (anemia) or low levels of folic acid (which can be detected with a simple blood test), the treatment is simply taking iron or folic acid supplements. For most people, however, medications are prescribed, such as carbidopa/levodopa (Sinemet), pramipexole (Mirapex), clonazepam (Klonopin), or temazepam (Restoril). In addition, it is known that caffeine makes RLS and PLMS much worse. Alcohol can also exacerbate symptoms. Therefore, cutting back or eliminating caffeine and alcohol may help. Finally, getting adequate sleep will also help, because sleep deprivation will make these problems worse.

One unusual and disturbing situation associated with RLS and PLMS is that the medications for these disorders often make other sleep disorders worse. For example, Klonopin, while it may solve the RLS or PLMS problem, will make sleep apnea worse. In turn, the treatments for many other sleep disorders often make RLS or PLMS worse. If an antidepressant is prescribed to alleviate narcolepsy, for example, it can make PLMS worse. It is therefore important that a person's sleep disorders be diagnosed and that the proper combination of treatments be utilized.

NARCOLEPSY

David is thirty-eight years old. He is always sleepy. Even as far back as the ninth grade he remembers falling asleep in class on a regular basis. He is afraid to drive because he has already had one near accident from falling asleep at the wheel. His wife and his boss are frustrated with him because he keeps falling asleep. The other day he even fell asleep in the middle of an important meeting with a new client.

David has narcolepsy, a relatively rare disorder that can significantly interfere with a person's ability to function. Although there is no "cure" for narcolepsy, it can be treated, and people with this disorder can lead normal lives.

Narcolepsy usually begins during adolescence, although there have been documented cases of its occurring before puberty. Symptoms can appear suddenly or can develop slowly over years.

Narcolepsy is often referred to as "sleeping sickness," although the way it is often portrayed on television, with someone constantly falling asleep whether standing up, sitting down, or even while playing baseball, is not correct.

Symptoms of Narcolepsy

There are four major symptoms of narcolepsy, although not everyone with narcolepsy has all of these symptoms.

1. **Excessive daytime sleepiness.** Daytime sleepiness is usually the first symptom, and for some people the only symptom, of narcolepsy. People with narcolepsy may feel sleepy all the time or just frequently throughout the day. They may feel sleepy at times that other people feel sleepy, such as after a heavy meal or during a boring lecture, but they also feel sleepy at those times when normal people wouldn't, such as during an exciting movie, while talking on the telephone, or while driving. If a person with narcolepsy takes a short nap when feeling sleepy, he usually feels refreshed afterward.

2. **Cataplexy.** "Cataplexy" refers to brief episodes of sudden loss of muscle control. The feeling can be mild with just weakness in the knees, or it can be severe with complete loss of muscle control leading to a fall. Cataplexy is triggered by a strong emotion, such as laughter, surprise, anger, or anxiety. Some people have simply to think about an emotional event, and they will have cataplexy. Cataplexy only occurs with narcolepsy; that is, if someone has cataplexy, then he definitely has narcolepsy. Cataplexy can be the first symptom of narcolepsy or may develop years later, or not at all.

3. **Sleep paralysis.** This occurs when a person is waking up or falling asleep. It is a feeling that the person is unable to move or speak. Sleep paralysis usually lasts for only a few moments, but to the affected person it can feel endless. If the person is touched by another, the sleep paralysis will disappear. Some people refer to sleep paralysis as "witch riding," the belief that a witch is sitting on the person's chest. And while it may be associated with narcolepsy, many people who do not have narcolepsy experience sleep paralysis.

4. **Hypnagogic hallucinations.** These also occur when a person is waking up or falling asleep. These are dreamlike events that are difficult to distinguish from reality. The person is awake but is seeing or hearing images or sounds. Often these dreams are mistaken for the hallucinations of someone who is schizophrenic. People other than those with narcolepsy experience this phenomenon, especially when sleep deprived.

In addition to these four major symptoms, individuals with narcolepsy may also experience other symptoms.

1. **Automatic behavior.** This is the performance of routine tasks without the person's being aware of doing it. These activities can include such simple things as folding laundry or having a conversation. They can occur at times that are potentially dangerous, such as when driving a car or cooking. Sometimes the person does something inappropriate, such as putting dishes into the washing machine rather than the dishwasher. The person has no recollection of doing these automatic behaviors.

2. **Disturbed nighttime sleep.** Surprisingly, although individuals with narcolepsy may feel sleepy all day and even

have difficulty staying awake, their nighttime sleep may be disturbed. People with narcolepsy can wake frequently during the night, adding to the problem of their daytime sleepiness.

3. **Dreaming during naps.** Most people do not dream when taking a short nap, less than thirty minutes. Individuals with narcolepsy typically will dream. In addition, someone with narcolepsy finds a short nap refreshing, whereas others may feel groggy upon waking up.

4. **Impaired functioning.** Because of the excessive daytime sleepiness, many individuals with narcolepsy have impaired functioning; that is, they may feel lethargic all the time, be unable to concentrate at school or at work, and even have memory problems. Narcolepsy can definitely interfere with school or work performance, and it usually takes a toll on marriages and families if not diagnosed and treated.

What Causes Narcolepsy?

The exact cause of narcolepsy is still not known. The symptoms of narcolepsy apparently involve the regions of the central nervous system that control sleeping and waking. Many of these symptoms are caused by what is called "REM intrusion." As you may recall from Chapter 2, there are two major stages of sleep, non-REM and REM. REM sleep is characterized by dreaming and muscle paralysis. People with narcolepsy keep moving into REM sleep, as if their body doesn't get enough of it and needs more of it or because the central nervous system switch is unable to suppress REM sleep.

Recent discoveries suggest that the neurotransmitter orexin/ hypocretin is involved in narcolepsy. Some believe that autoimmune mechanisms combined with environmental factors are involved. Narcolepsy tends to run in families, indicating a potential genetic link. If someone is diagnosed with narcolepsy, there is often, although not always, a parent, grandparent, or aunt or uncle with the same problems, which may or may not have been diagnosed.

Treatment

As mentioned above, there is no known cure for narcolepsy. Instead, the treatment of narcolepsy focuses on managing the disorder in the following ways.

MEDICATION. Many people with narcolepsy try to treat themselves, often without realizing it, by ingesting large quantities of caffeine. There are some who will drink twelve cups of coffee, two liters of caffeinated Coke, or a gallon of iced tea in one day. Others will take over-the-counter medications such as Nō-Dōz. This system does not work well and can interfere with nighttime sleep, which doesn't help the daytime sleepiness.

A better method is developing a medication regimen with a physician. Medications can be given to decrease daytime sleepiness and to help control cataplexy. Two stimulant medications that are commonly prescribed for the daytime sleepiness are Cylert and Ritalin. Another stimulant medication that is used specifically for narcolepsy is Provigil. Drugs to control cataplexy include imipramine and desipramine. Although these medications are traditionally used as antidepressants, they are prescribed not because the person is depressed but because they suppress REM, the cause of cataplexy.

LIFESTYLE MANAGEMENT. Some changes in lifestyle may help individuals with narcolepsy control their disorder. The following suggestions are often extremely helpful:

+ *Get a good night's sleep.* This includes having a good sleep schedule. Go to bed and get up at the same time every day.
+ *Nap on a schedule.* Take one to two short naps every day to help feel alert and refreshed.

✦ *Avoid tasks or jobs that are repetitive or boring.* The more physical and active the job, the better.

✦ *Avoid driving or other dangerous activities,* such as swimming or riding a bicycle, when sleepy.

PROVIDE INFORMATION AND EDUCATE. It is very important that your family, friends, and coworkers know and understand your narcolepsy. Do not try to hide it, as others will notice, and rather than attribute your sleepiness to a sleep disorder, they will often believe that you are lazy, bored, insolent, or depressed. Some will even think that you have a psychiatric or psychological problem. So be sure to inform people. If your adolescent has narcolepsy, make sure that all teachers are informed and educated.

SEEK SUPPORT FROM A SUPPORT GROUP. There are many others out there who also have narcolepsy. See Appendix B for resources that will help you find a local support group in your area. If one isn't available, start one.

Reminders

✦ Sleep disorders are experienced by 25–30 percent of all adults.

✦ A thorough assessment of sleep disorders will include an extensive interview concerning sleep patterns, the maintenance of a sleep diary, and possibly an overnight polysomnography.

✦ Insomnia involves difficulty falling asleep or maintaining sleep. It can have many different causes but is highly treatable.

✦ Snoring is a common sleep disorder that can disrupt your sleep and the sleep of others.

✦ Sleep apnea involves repetitive pauses in breathing during sleep and can be dangerous to your health.

✦ Restless legs syndrome and periodic limb movements in sleep can interfere with going to sleep and can lead to frequent wakings throughout the night.

✦ Narcolepsy, a rare disorder, involves excessive daytime sleepiness and other unusual symptoms.

✦ There are more than eighty diagnosed sleep disorders, with the most common ones discussed here. Don't allow a sleep problem suffered by you or someone in your family to go undiagnosed and untreated. Seek help and get treatment so that everyone gets a good night's sleep.

Appendices

Baby Bedtime Books

BOOKS FOR INFANTS

Animal Crackers: Bedtime, Jane Dyer
   A board book collection of classic bedtime lullabies.

A Child's Good Night Book, Margaret Wise Brown
   In this award-winning story, sheep, kangaroos, bunnies, and children all
   close their eyes and go to sleep.

The Going to Bed Book, Sandra Boynton
   A silly book about animals going to bed on a boat. Very enjoyable.

Good Night, Baby, Clara Vulliamy
   A lullaby book about bedtime for a baby.

Good Night Gorilla, Peggy Rathmann
   A gorilla and all the other animals sneak out of the zoo at bedtime to all
   get in bed with the zookeeper's wife.

Goodnight Moon, Margaret Wise Brown
   Goodnight Moon is the all-time classic book for bedtime. Many parents
   say that this is the first book they ever read to their baby at bedtime.

Hush Little Baby, Sylvia Long
   A wonderful version of the classic children's lullaby.

Maybe, My Baby, Marilyn Janovitz
   Animal parents and their little ones cuddle to sleep.

Night, Night, Mark Burgess
   A rhyming book about a bear's getting ready for bed.

One Sleepy Baby, Pamela Levin
A wonderful book that counts down to bedtime for baby, starting with one sleepy baby and two tired eyes.

Pajama Time! Sandra Boynton
An enjoyable story about pajamas and getting ready for bed.

Pat the Bunny: Sleepy Bunny, Golden Books
A cloth book that has a toy bunny that your baby can help get ready for bed.

Sleep Rhymes from Around the World, Jane Yolen
A wonderful collection of lullabies from around the world.

Ten Bears in a Bed, John Richardson
A classic counting rhyme about ten bears in a bed, based on the children's song "Roll Over." This edition is a delightful pop-up book.

BOOKS FOR TODDLERS

Bedtime, Everybody, Mordicai Gerstein
A little girl, Daisy, tries to get her stuffed animals to go to bed.

Bedtime for Frances, Russell Hoban
Frances, the beloved bear, uses well-known stalling tactics at bedtime.

Dr. Seuss's Sleep Book, Dr. Seuss
A favorite Dr. Seuss story about sleep, where everyone is yawning.

Five Little Monkeys Jumping on the Bed, Eileen Christelow
Five little monkeys get ready for bed. This book is a remake of the classic children's song.

Good Night, Copycub, Richard Edwards
Copycub's mother tells him a story to help him fall asleep.

How Do Dinosaurs Say Good Night? Jane Yolen and Mark Teague
An entertaining story of how dinosaurs say good night. They don't stomp their feet or put up a fight. They turn out the light and give a big hug, of course.

How Many Kisses Do You Want Tonight? Varsha Bajaj
> Parents ask their baby animals, "How many kisses do you want tonight?"
> A wonderful and warm bedtime ritual.

I Am Not Sleepy and I Will Not Go to Bed, Lauren Child
> Charlie, a big brother, tries to get his sister Lola to bed. A funny and
> imaginative book for the older toddler and preschooler.

The Napping House, Audrey Wood
> A story in cumulative rhyme about a house where everyone is sleeping,
> including a snoozing cat, a dozing dog, and a dreaming child.

The Noisy Way to Bed, Ian Whybrow
> A little boy wants to go to bed but a duck, a horse, a sheep, and a pig
> won't let him. All end up in bed together.

Sailing Off to Sleep, Linda Ashman
> A little girl imagines wonderful adventures rather than going to bed, but
> realizes that she really is ready for bed.

Sleep Tight, Little Mouse, Mary Morgan
> Little Mouse can't fall asleep but realizes the best place to be is at home
> with his mother.

Sleep Well, Little Bear, Quint Buchholz
> A little bear who can't fall asleep thinks about his day and makes plans
> for the next, until he is ready to go to sleep.

Sleepy Bears, Mem Fox
> Mother Bear tells each of her six cubs a special rhyme to help them drift
> off to sleep.

Time for Bed, Mem Fox
> This book says good night to all the animals.

When Mama Comes Home Tonight, Eileen Spinelli
> A lovely story for working mothers on the special rituals shared when a
> parent comes home from work.

The Yawn Heard 'Round the World, Scott Thomas
> A little girl claims that she's not sleepy, but then her yawn makes a jour-
> ney around the world.

BOOKS FOR DEALING WITH BEDTIME FEARS

Go Away Big Green Monster, Ed Emberley
This award-winning book helps children deal with their nighttime fears.

It's Bedtime, Brigitte Weninger
A little boy rejects all of his cuddly stuffed toys to sleep with and chooses instead a scary monster doll who will keep him safe and scare away all the other monsters and ghosts.

My Mama Says There Aren't Any Zombies, Ghosts, Vampires, Creatures, Demons, Monsters, Fiends, Goblins, or Things, Judith Viorst
Although a little boy's mother insists that none of these things exist, he is not so sure.

There's an Alligator Under My Bed, Mercer Mayer
A boy bravely confronts the alligator that lives under his bed, one that no one else can see.

There's a Nightmare in My Closet, Mercer Mayer
A little boy discovers that the nightmare in his closet is just as scared as he is.

We're Going on a Bear Hunt, Michael Rosen and Helen Oxenbury
This children's classic is about a family going on a bear hunt insisting, "We're not scared," only to return to the safety of their bed.

Where the Wild Things Are, Maurice Sendak
A boy confronts the scary things that appear in his dreams.

Resources for Parents

PRODUCTS

Crib tent. A mesh crib tent will keep your baby in the crib and will not allow him to climb out. It attaches with Velcro to the top of the crib rails. A crib tent keeps a little one snug and safe. It also keeps pets out. Crib tents attach to any standard-size crib.

Crib sheets. Crib sheets attach to the bars of the crib with Velcro, making sheet changing much easier. Many stores and online Web sites that specialize in baby items carry these sheets.

Stores/Web sites

The following stores carry baby items, including the above products:

Babies "R" Us
www.babiesrus.com

Baby Center Store
www.babycenter.com

One Step Ahead
(800)274-8440
www.onestepahead.com

ORGANIZATIONS AND ASSOCIATIONS

General Sleep

American Academy of Sleep Medicine
One Westbrook Corporate Center
Suite 920
Westchester, IL 60154
(708)492-0930
www.aasmnet.com

> The American Academy of Sleep Medicine is a professional membership organization dedicated to the advancement of sleep medicine. This organization accredits sleep centers. You can find on their Web site a listing of accredited sleep centers in your area. It also has a number of educational materials available.

Sleep Research Society
One Westbrook Corporate Center
Suite 920
Westchester, IL 60154
(708)492-0930
www.sleepresearchsociety.org

> The Sleep Research Society is a professional membership organization dedicated to the advancement of academic sleep medicine, fostering research and scientific investigation.

National Sleep Foundation
1522 K Street, NW
Suite 500
Washington, DC 20005
(202)347-3471
www.sleepfoundation.org

> The National Sleep Foundation is a nonprofit organization dedicated to improving public health and safety by achieving understanding of sleep and sleep disorders, and by supporting education, sleep-related research, and advocacy.

Sleep Apnea

American Sleep Apnea Association (ASAA)
1424 K Street, NW
Suite 302
Washington, DC 20005
(202)293-3656
www.sleepapnea.org

> The ASAA is an organization dedicated to promoting education and awareness of sleep apnea. The ASAA AWAKE is a network of support groups throughout the United States. In addition, they publish a newsletter entitled *Wake up Call: The Wellness Letter for Snoring and Apnea* and have information regarding sleep apnea available on their Web site.

Restless Legs

Restless Legs Syndrome Foundation, Inc.
819 Second Street, SW
Rochester, MN 55902
(507)287-6465
www.rls.org

> The RLS Foundation's mission is to increase awareness of restless legs syndrome, to improve treatments, and to support research. Their Web site provides comprehensive information on RLS and contact information for local support groups.

Narcolepsy

Narcolepsy Network, Inc.
10921 Reed Hartman Highway, Suite 119
Cincinnati, OH 45242
(513)891-3836
www.narcolepsynetwork.org

> The Narcolepsy Network is a resource center to facilitate support groups, provide public education, and encourage ongoing scientific research in sleep medicine.

SIDS

National SIDS/Infant Death Resource Center
2070 Chain Bridge Road, Suite 450
Vienna, VA 22182
(866)866-7437
www.sidscenter.org

SIDS Alliance
1314 Bedford Avenue
Suite 210
Baltimore, MD 21208
(410)653-8226
www.sidsalliance.com

Twins and More Groups

Mainly Multiples
941 Matthews-Mint Hill
Suite M
Matthews, NC 28105
(800)388-TWIN
www.morethan1.com
    Distributes a catalog of products available for twins.

National Organization of Mothers of Twins Clubs (NOMOTC)
PO Box 438
Thompsons Station, TN 37179
(877)540-2200
www.nomotc.com
    A nationwide network of parents of multiples clubs that share information and advice.

Mothers of Supertwins
PO Box 306
East Islip, NY 11730
(631)859-1110
www.mostonline.org
    A support and information network for parents of triplets, quadruplets, and more.

Breast-feeding

La Leche League International
1400 North Meacham Road
Schaumburg, IL 60173-4808
(847)519-7730
(800)525-3243
www.lalecheleague.org

General Parenting Web sites

BabyCenter.com and ParentCenter.com
Child.com
Parents.com
Parenting.com

Index